CONCEIVABLE

A Guide to Making 2SLGBTQ+ Family

CONCEIVABLE

A Guide to Making 2SLGBTQ+ Family

Written and Collected by Laine Halpern Zisman

Illustrated by Kelsy Vivash

FERNWOOD PUBLISHING
HALIFAX & WINNIPEG

Development editing: Tanya Andrusieczko and Jazz Cook
Copyediting: Jenn Harris
Cover design and Illustrations: Kelsy Vivash
Design and layout: Lauren Jeanneau
Printed and bound in Canada

Published by Fernwood Publishing
Halifax and Winnipeg
2970 Oxford Street, Halifax, Nova Scotia, B3L 2W4
fernwoodpublishing.ca

Fernwood Publishing Company Limited gratefully acknowledges the financial
support of the Government of Canada through the Canada Book Fund and
the Canada Council for the Arts. We acknowledge the Province of Manitoba
for support through the Manitoba Publishers Marketing Assistance Program
and the Book Publishing Tax Credit. We acknowledge the Province of Nova
Scotia through the Publishers Assistance Fund.

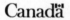 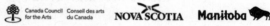 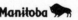

Library and Archives Canada Cataloguing in Publication
Title: Conceivable : a guide to making 2SLGBTQ+ family / written and
collected by Laine Halpern Zisman, M.A., PhD ; illustrated by Kelsy Vivash.
Names: Halpern Zisman, Laine, author.
Description: Includes bibliographical references and index.
Identifiers: Canadiana (print) 20240434846 | Canadiana (ebook) 20240437594
| ISBN 9781773636894 (softcover) | ISBN 9781773636986 (EPUB)
Subjects: LCSH: Sexual minority parents—Canada. | LCSH: Sexual minorities'
families—Canada. | LCSH: Family planning—Canada. | LCSH: Fertility,
Human—Canada. | LCSH: Conception.
Classification: LCC HQ73.63.C3 .H35 2024 | DDC 306.85086/60971—dc23

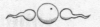

Contents

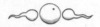

Acronyms and Initialisms

2SLGBTQ+	Two-spirit, lesbian, gay, bisexual, trans, queer +
AFC	antral follicle count
AHRA	Assisted Human Reproduction Act
AIDS	acquired immunodeficiency syndrome
AMH	anti-Müllerian hormone
ART	assisted reproductive technology
BBT	basal body temperature
BIPOC	Black, Indigenous, people of colour
CMV	cytomegalovirus
D&C	dilation and curettage
FE-SET	frozen euploid single embryo transfers
FHA	functional hypothalamic amenorrhea
FSH	follicle-stimulating hormone
GAHT	gender-affirming hormone therapy
GnRH	gonadotropin-releasing hormone
HCG	human chorionic gonadotropin
HIV	human immunodeficiency virus
HPO	hypothalamus, pituitary, and ovaries (axis of)
ICI	intracervical insemination
ICSI	intracytoplasmic sperm injection
IUI	intrauterine insemination

IVF	in vitro fertilization
LH	luteinizing hormone
MVA	manual vacuum aspiration
PIO	progesterone in oil
PCOS	polycystic ovary syndrome
PGT-A	preimplantation genetic testing for aneuploidy
PGT-M	preimplantation genetic testing for monogenic disorders
PMADS	perinatal or postpartum mood and anxiety disorder
PTSD	post-traumatic stress disorder
REI	reproductive endocrinologist
RIVF	reciprocal in vitro fertilization
STI	sexually transmitted infection
TTC	trying to conceive
TWW	two-week wait

For Joanna, Tybilee, and Percy
Let's build a beautiful, wild world together

Introduction

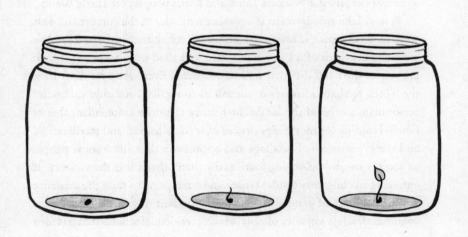

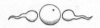

AN ACKNOWLEDGEMENT OF THE LAND

I am writing from my home in Toronto, also known as Tkaronto. This land has been the home and hunting ground for many peoples, including the Haudenosaunee, Anishinaabe, Wendat, Cree, and the Mississaugas of the Credit, as well as all other caretakers of this land, acknowledged and unacknowledged, recorded and unrecorded. This territory is bound by the Dish with One Spoon agreement between the Haudenosaunee Confederacy and the Ojibwe and allied nations to peaceably share and care for the resources around the Great Lakes. In writing and collecting contributions for this book, I recognize the ongoing impact of settler colonialism on family and kinship for Indigenous Peoples and the enduring presence and rights of all First Nations, Inuit, and Métis peoples on Turtle Island.

A land acknowledgement is a present reminder of the current and past ways in which space is colonized, occupied, cohabited, and cared for. We wear the histories of a space like a skin and shed our stories with each particle of dust and dirt that falls in our wake. Even when we don't have the words to share a history or memories to recall it, our physical bodies accumulate stories of the land. The history of settler colonialism shapes family building journeys, experiences of medicalization and sterilization, and the experiences of privilege and oppression that allow some people to access care and belonging more easily than others. It is the violence of enforcing an obligatory gender binary and attempting to erase the existence of a multiplicity of gender experiences and identities across Indigenous communities. It is a history of genocide and residential schools that has torn families apart and cut the branches and roots of family trees. It is how past and current sterilization and violence prohibit Indigenous Peoples from safely accessing care and impede their ability to build equitable family supports. It is the lived fear and pain that results from evacuation policies that take Indigenous Peoples outside of their communities to birth their babies without community, family, or other supports. A land acknowledgement in the context of this book is about facing the ongoing ways in which conception, birth, and life are shaped by a colonial and white supremacist project and the barriers that create health disparities for many Indigenous Peoples in this country.

WHO AM I? FROM THIS LITTLE JAR

I am an Ashkenazi third-generation Holocaust survivor whose maternal family — may their memories be a blessing — was nearly wiped out by murder at the hands of Hitler and the Nazi regime. The roots of my family tree are grounded in memories of people who died too young for who they are. I am a settler with white skin, a cisgender woman, a wife of a wife, and a mother. I am a second-generation queer person, with a mother who taught me that sexual orientation means more than the partner you are with. My own journeys through relationships, family building, parenthood, and understanding of self have been shaped by the historical and current experiences of my communities and my kin.

My grandmother survived unimaginable terrors of genocide and was the sole survivor in her family. She would often speak of how important it was to her to continue her story, to extend the roots to our family tree. She used to look at all of us sitting around the family dinner table, eyes wide and in awe. "From this little jar," she would say, gesturing to herself and opening her arms wide to all of us. New worlds are birthed from our matriarchs and elders. *From this little jar.* I learn from her what love and acceptance can be: the importance of family, lineage, and kinship, whatever that might look like, whatever form that might take. May each of us continue the legacy of our elders, from their little jars to our future worlds, generations of love, support, and compassionate kinship.

This is not your typical "how to make a baby" book and I do not provide any medical advice in it. I am not a physician, a reproductive endocrinologist (REI), or a nurse. I am a researcher, a certified full spectrum doula, and a fertility support practitioner. While writing this book, I am also completing a postdoctoral fellowship at the School of Public Health and Social Policy at the University of Victoria in British Columbia, doing research on 2SLGBTQ+ health equity. I bring all of my experience working with clients, researching, and supporting community into the pages of this book. This is a guide, a companion, an expansion of communities, and — I hope — an invitation to be a companion to yourself in this journey.

WHO IS THIS BOOK FOR?

This book is for *you*. This book is for people who are trying to build families in a world that often doesn't make space for them. Some of us are queer, some are trans, some are asexual, some are co-parenting, and some are single parents by choice. This book is also for you if your queer or chosen family member is choosing to have a baby and you are working to educate yourself. If your partner, friend, parent, or other relation is thinking about having a baby: this book is for you too. If you are looking for a donor, considering becoming a donor, are just curious about the politics and regulations for 2SLGBTQ+ family building in

Canada, this book is for you too. This book is for you, whether you fall within the acronym of 2SLGBTQ+ or somewhere outside of its identities and communities. The "you" I refer to throughout this book is a fluid signifier for all the people navigating a not-so-mainstream family-building journey and seeking access to information and resources, people who need and deserve answers to their questions. Sometimes, the "you" I refer to will resonate with your needs and experiences, and sometimes it might not quite apply to your specific experiences. For whatever reason you picked up this book, I hope you find a place in these pages. This book is for all of us who are absent from the baby-making narratives or the idealized image of the white picket fence.

This book is also an invitation to connect with yourself on this family-building journey, to figure out what you want and ways to communicate those needs, and to understand the politics, the challenges, and the opportunities for agency and joy on this journey. This book offers insights and ideas on different ways to pursue reproduction and the ways that our identities and experiences might shape our fertility journeys. In Canada, there are policies that both protect and hinder 2SLGBTQ+ reproduction. Some of these policies are written into law and some of them are a result of activities or guidelines at fertility clinics or doctors' offices. It is important that we understand our rights and that we know what questions to ask in order to avoid unnecessary barriers to achieving our goals.

The community members, specialists, and contributors to this book come from many backgrounds and fields. They offer their first-hand experiences and knowledge as doulas, researchers, lawyers, and care practitioners to direct you towards resources and help you to ask the right questions. Each experience will be different and there is no catch-all solution or approach to building a family. But knowledge is essential to advocacy and community building, and this journey is made easier through educated collaboration, supportive collectivity, and revolutionary growth.

WHO IS IN OUR CONVERSATION?

This book is part of a conversation. We decide together who we want to bring to the table: Who is this book a companion to? What other information are you seeking, and what information do you need to know more generally? I think of this text as a roadmap to help you get where you are going, but I hope it is also a choose-your-own-adventure. There are books that live on my shelf, on my bedside table, in my bathroom, that are companions. I pick them up and turn the pages looking for where to begin (a first page is never *the* first page). I skim the pages looking for poetry that moves me, words I need to hear, answers to questions. I hope this book is your companion too. You don't need to read it straight through from beginning to end. You don't have to read it in order. I promise it will not have every answer to each of your questions. But I hope it helps you to find your voice to ask the questions you need to ask.

I've invited people formally into the conversation — they have shared their ideas in the pages of this book, and I will share resources with you for texts, rituals, and practices that might be useful in your journey. And I am inviting you into the conversation too. We are creating it together. I remember fumbling through the pages of books about bodies and vulvas and menstruation that my mother lovingly bought for me as I developed and how they welcomed me to share my own experiences within the lines of the text. I loved having a chance to reflect, to write, and to question and I still return to those pages today. So, I hope this book looks nothing like this book by the time you have moved through the pages. Fill the margins of these pages with curiosity. Ask questions, draw pictures, trace the outline of your fingertips, syringes, and vitamins. Make a memory from ovulation strips, sperm test results, or questions for a donor. Write a letter to your future family and imagine their voices as they read and reread their stories. Tear, fold, write, doodle, draw, crumple, ask this book to be what other books are not: *messy*.

This book is organized in nine parts that aim to prepare you and your family for the family-building process. The first three parts focus on setting the foundation for your journey, understanding context and history, and building your community support networks for this process. Parts 4 to 7 deal with core "how-to" topics to help you understand all the options that may be available to you and offer tools for making big decisions or navigating change if your plan doesn't go as you imagined. The last two parts are about transitions. Part 8 looks at the experience of loss and grief that are part of some people's family-building journeys, including what to expect from a miscarriage and strategies for moving through grief and mourning. The final part looks at what might come after this book ends, along with the transitions some families make into parenthood. Throughout the book there are contributions from others working in the field — doulas, lawyers, nurses — who provide their unique insights and perspective on 2SLGBTQ+ fertility and reproductive journeys. There are also activities and prompts in each part that you can reflect on when they resonate with you.

One of the goals of this book is to remind you that *you* are part of this journey — you are part of this conversation — whatever role you might take. Your body might be one that helps to create a baby with sperm or eggs. Your body might be a body that will carry a baby as a parent or as a surrogate. Your body might feed a baby upon their arrival, with your body or with a bottle full of nourishing food. Your body might be one that rocks a future baby or waves to them. Your body might be one that models consent and asks for a hug. Your body might be far away, reaching through a video call to sing lullabies and teach words. Building our families looks different to each of us. But for each of us it is shaped by our experience in our bodies, the histories that mark our bodies, and the spaces our bodies take up. I hope you can read this book in spaces where you feel expansive, welcome, and full. I hope this book can help you in the process of finding these spaces and making these spaces.

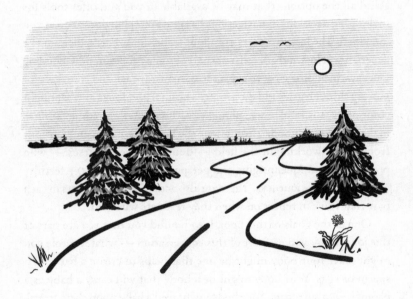

1.
Expanding
Your Family

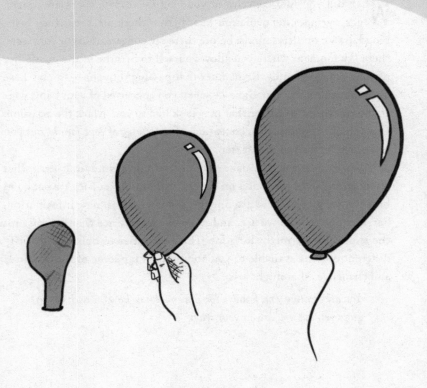

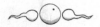

This first part is about situating yourself in this journey and learning
how you might use this book. It is a big-picture overview of what
to expect when you want to be expecting. Read it if you are thinking about starting or growing your family, already in the process of
building it, or have questions about what to expect from this text.

When did you first conceive of your family? Before there are sperm,
eggs, syringes, or ovulation kits; before there are pregnancy tests,
blood draws, or ultrasounds; before there are conversations or contracts;
there is a moment where you allow yourself to breathe in the possibility
of your growing family. Remember that passing thought — it may have
been momentous or mundane — when you conceived of your baby, your
changing family, whatever that may look like to you. Mark the occasion.
It is only the beginning of conception, of *conceiving of your family*, but you
can celebrate it as your first step.

There is no one way to make a baby or to build a family and often what
we imagine will be the routes on our family-building journey are not quite
how we get there. There are unexpected challenges, new information,
barriers due to who we are, and policies and politics that can disrupt
the simplicity we might long for. This book tries to help you identify
different options available to you and prepare for some of the obstacles
and challenges that might arise.

*You are creating your family. You may not know how (or with whom)
quite yet, but you are on your way.*

In her book *Queering Reproduction*, Laura Mamo reminds us: "Nothing within biology demands the nuclear family" (2007: 5). The Western heteronormative idea of family is geographically, historically, and culturally specific. "Family" has not always been the fantasy of two cisgender, heterosexual parents and 1.5 kids behind a white picket fence. Expanding family is also about expanding our *ideas* of family. You are building your family whether or not you already have a baby, whether or not you co-parent, adopt, or bring furry friends into the mix. Your family is not determined by a baby or if you choose to have one at all. A baby does not make a family. *You do.*

Queering family means that one person can be a family or a dozen people can be a family. We define our terms, and they can be fluid, flexible, and changing. This book focuses on some ways to build your family, some ways to try to conceive (TTC), some ways to think about the people who might be involved in your child-rearing, growth, and transformations of learning, parenting, and building relationships. But these are not the only way. Queer theory and queer experience teach us to live *otherwise*. What does that mean? We don't need to adhere their norms.

FOUR TRUTHS ABOUT FAMILY BUILDING

Four things often come up in my work with 2SLGBTQ+ intended families. These "four truths" may resonate with your experience or they might fall short. After reading these pages, I encourage you to write values, priorities, or truths that resonate with your experience right now. The activity at the end of Part 1 offers questions to help you identify the values that you are leading with at this stage of your journey. You can return to these pages in a few weeks, months, or years and share how these truths have transformed or changed.

Truth 1. Your Journey Has Already Begun

As 2SLGBTQ+ intended parents, our journey often begins well before our "first try." We spend months contemplating, researching, reaching out, on waitlists, with doctors. And in all of these steps we exert energy, labour, and emotions and often don't feel empowered to say we are "trying to conceive." We feel like we need an egg, sperm, uterus, ovulation before we have the freedom to say we are *really* trying. This mindset can be disempowering and invalidating. You are on this journey, you have started this journey, whenever those words feel right to you. The work you are putting in now is part of your family's conception story. This is it. You are doing it. Your journey has already begun.

Truth 2. Expect the Unexpected

One thing I find myself saying again and again is to expect the unexpected. Every day, week, month, every hour, will bring with it new learnings, new surprises, and new emotional shifts. We want strategy, a plan, step-by-step instructions on what comes next and sometimes we are fortunate enough to get just that: a seamless point A to point B baby-making experience without hiccups or obstacles. But for most of us, that is not the case. Surprises are part of this process — a shift in ovulation date, a donor too busy to come to your home, an unanticipated need for medical intervention — we cannot guess what is to come, but we can prepare ourselves with strategies to cope with change. I hope this book offers you the opportunity to build those skills.

Truth 3. You Are Stronger with Your "Team"

The truth about family building is that we need teams, we need community, and we need you. We need to remember that the technical stuff, the first steps, the next steps, and the medications, the conversations are all just the beginning, even when they feel like an end. Your team, your chosen family, your expanded network, your doctors, providers, caregivers, aunties, friends, non-human furry companions, your books, your music, your creations, your inspirations — you need them all. Your team is alive and shifting. They are the people and things that make you feel in good company. You will need them now as you begin, and you will need them as you navigate pregnancy and parenthood. You will need them as advocates, tender ears to listen, people to scream, rage, and celebrate with. You will need your team. We don't need to do this alone.

Truth 4. Oppression and Inequity Impact 2SLGBTQ+ Fertility Care

While access to equitable healthcare is a fundamental right that should be extended to all people in this country, implicit and explicit discrimination against 2SLGBTQ+ communities, both individually and systemically, often impacts the services and support they receive in Canada. The language used by staff and doctors, limitations of electronic medical records, and a lack of 2SLGBTQ+ training can all impact 2SLGBTQ+ access to quality healthcare (Comeau et al., 2023). Comeau et al. note that only 10 percent of medical students felt prepared to care for transgender patients. This may be because only one-third of medical schools in North America provide education on hormone therapy and surgical transition (Comeau et al. 2023: 119). A lack of knowledge can lead to a lack of care. In their survey of emergency medicine physicians and residents, Lien et al. (2021) note that 54 percent of respondents had witnessed discriminatory comments about 2SLGBTQ+ patients or staff and 21 percent of respondents described having less eye contact with 2SLGBTQ+ patients at least some of the time. *Less eye contact: the realization and materialization of being unseen.* We know that micro- and macroaggressions impact who can and will access care, their health outcomes, and their physical and mental health. One of the main objectives of this book is to name systems of oppression, identify gaps in medical training, and help families navigate systems that weren't made for them.

In their chapter, "Creating Community and Creating Family: Our QTBIPOC Parenting Group," Audrey Dwyer, a Toronto-based queer artist and activist, shares the need for queer and trans family-building spaces that do not just teach tools or processes for reproductive journeys, but also the politics of family building. When they couldn't find an existing group to fit their needs, they created their own, gathering as a collective in their homes to talk, to share, to eat, and to build community. Dwyer writes:

> Due to colonization and white supremacy, we queers have so much to push against. We try to work through all of these obstacles while building community and nourishing people ... we wanted to deal with more emotionally rooted, chal-lenging issues in a way that respected and took care of our humanity with dignity. Building community is an intentional thing, and our group is rooted in intention. (2018: 234)

Being silenced, not feeling heard, or being unable to voice your needs because of fear of repercussions are products of systemic power struc-tures and oppression. We don't feel we can speak up when we (and our communities) have been silenced or ignored historically and currently. Building community and finding or creating spaces for support are often crucial while navigating the healthcare system, advocating for dignity, and demanding to be seen.

Gentle Encouragement

Not everyone has the same experience trying to build their families. Sometimes being happy, being excited, being hopeful is the most vulnerable state you can be. However, I offer the following as a reminder for a future you or a permission slip for your current self: You don't have to be happy or excited or hopeful. You can be scared. You can be overwhelmed. You can be anxious. As your mixed and confusing emotions come up, your job is to acknowledge them.

Whether you are trying to create your family at home, with a donor, at a clinic, through a surrogate, with partner(s), on your own, or with co-parents, *you* are an integral part of this process. One of the ways we can feel disempowered, dysregulated, and out of control is when you lose yourself in the story. This is happening with and to *you* — regardless of the specific role you are playing in your family. Doctors and healthcare practitioners can sometimes make us feel like a number with a blanket protocol. We are ticking boxes, a check on a to-do list: a sperm analysis, a signature on a form, an intrauterine insemination (IUI), or an egg retrieval. Even the most well-meaning doctor can have too much on their plate and hustle you through an appointment, without time to reflect on information shared or pause for questions or opportunities for learning. And in all of the steps we have to take, in all of the long list of decisions, scheduling, worries, and celebrations, finding gametes, preparing our bodies, or supporting the bodies who will carry, *we sometimes forget to support ourselves.*

Name It to Tame It

Daniel Siegel (1999), a psychiatrist, writer, and professor, created a simple technique called "Name It to Tame It" to help the body and brain snap out of a fight/flight/freeze response. In this simple practice, the act of naming how we are feeling can reset and regulate the system. When you name your emotions, you also create distance between you and the reaction you are having: you are not defined by your anxiety, you are experiencing it. If you find it helpful and safe, when intense emotions arise, follow these steps: take a few deep, slow breaths. When you feel ready, label the feelings, fears, or anxieties you're experiencing (for example: helpless, scared, angry, sad). Pay attention to your body's signals as you continue to breathe slowly and deeply. You can keep naming those feelings until you feel more regulated.

You Are Feeling Overwhelmed, Scared, or Anxious

Right now, you are allowed to feel scared. Right now, you are allowed to feel stressed. This experience is hard, and you are allowed to feel this deeply hard and painful feeling. Maybe today sucks. Give yourself a hug and take a breath. If there is a part of you that feels sad, talk to that part of you: "It's okay to feel sad. I am here with you." Sit with the part of you that is feeling hard feelings and keep it company. Let it know that it is allowed to be scared. Take another breath. A deep breath. Remind yourself that it is okay to cry or okay to scream or punch a pillow. If there is something that would feel good right now (going for a walk, taking a bath, having some tea), give that a try. Remember: this feeling right now is so hard. This part is so hard. This feeling will not be forever.

Take another deep breath.

USE THIS SPACE TO REFLECT ON YOUR FEELINGS

_____

_____

_____

_____

_____

_____

_____

_____

_____

_____

_____

_____

_____

_____

_____

_____

_____

_____

SOLO PARENTING, CO-PARENTING, PARTNER PARENTING

We know that all families look different. Some parents live in the same city together, some live across geographies, some are in romantic relationships, some are friends, and some are couples. Some families have four or five parents raising a child, some incorporate donor siblings (or diblings), and others allow their children to choose if they reach out to donor siblings in the future. Choosing a non-conventional family structure means that you are often "outed" or experience otherness in new ways than when you were not a parent or trying to grow your family. You are building a family in a system that was not designed for you. A paradox of visibility: you are at once erased, not easily found on forms, in doctor's offices, in books. But you are also hyper-visible, surveilled, questioned, too present, too seen.

Whether you are a solo parent, a multi-parent or poly family, co-parenting with a friend, or a queer or transgender dyad, you may feel like you don't fit. We have to cope with being everywhere and nowhere, and that can be complicated by our identities, family structures, and how easily we fit into the norms and expectations of our societies. It is … *exhausting*.

The tools and supports you need will depend on who you are, what you find comfort in, and the structure of your family. If you are co-parenting, look into laws and regulations regarding custody and parenthood. This is essential and will require legal intervention to ensure everyone's intentions and rights are clear, because all parents deserve to maintain their rights, regardless of how relationships and communication may change in your future. Sometimes, advocacy means making space for a family that does not fit neatly into the boxes on a form. If you are in a platonic co-parenting arrangement, you are not a known donor but a parent. Look into provincial fertility funding for cycle monitoring, IUI, and IVF (in vitro fertilization) and explore how it applies to donors, platonic co-parents, or partners. While provincial healthcare coverage often does *not* cover the cost of donor procedures or testing, the coverage may be less clear in platonic co-parenting arrangements.

Whether we are parenting alone, with multiple partners, or with non-romantic co-parents, our relationships are integral to building our families. There is no "good" or "better" or "secure" family attachment. There are just possibilities and opportunities for relationships, attachment, and security. Whoever you choose to go on this journey with, whatever your relationship shifts and turns into, know that your family is the right family for you and your humans.

Letter to a Non-gestational Parent

Dear non-gestational parent,

Hi, how are you? I hope you have been reading these pages and thinking and imagining the human(s) you will one day meet. This is your family and I know sometimes that can feel like the most exciting and thrilling thing in the world and other times you might have complicated feelings about how to support a gestational parent or feel helpless or detached from the process.

Your needs and voice matter. Don't be afraid to set boundaries, to be vulnerable and to talk about your fears, excitement, joys, and breaking points. It all matters. Set up times for conversations. What rituals, activities, or conversations will help you to continue to feel connected? The communication strategies you set up now are a foundation for your future and they will continue to grow and change and develop as you parent with your partner(s). The work you are all doing now will count for something. Your role is under-researched, not quite understood, and not perfectly supported. The mental health challenges you may encounter are wildly underserved, misunderstood, and sometimes invalidated. That does not mean that they are not valid. Being a non-gestational parent is a unique experience. All families look different. This book is for you too and you are part of this process. Keep checking in with yourself about your needs, your hopes, and how you want to be involved and connected to this process. You are both a support person for your partner(s) and a person who needs support. Congratulations on starting this journey and building your family. You got this!

ACTIVITY

• • •

YOUR TRUTHS ABOUT FAMILY BUILDING: LEADING WITH YOUR VALUES

Pause and remind yourself about you, your values, and your priorities. Reflect on what family building means to you. All parents involved in the journey can do this activity on their own and afterward share your insights with each other, listening to the other person and thinking about how you can stay communicative, connected, and present for each other. If you are a solo parent, consider sharing this with a friend, support person, or doula. Having the opportunity to talk about your values and get excited about your priorities and preferences can help us to find stability and validate that our choices are right for us. You can come back to your answers in months and years from now and consider how they have shifted, if they continue to reflect your values. What has changed, what have you learned?

Consider the following questions:

1. What motivates me in trying to build my family? What driving force moves me?

    _____

    _____

    _____

2. What beliefs (cultural, religious, community, personal) shape my views on starting or growing a family?

    _____

    _____

3. What cultural or community practices, religious or spiritual activities, or personal rituals do I imagine doing at each stage of this process: conception, birth, postpartum, parenting milestones?

    _____

    _____

    _____

4. How do I envision my family, parenting, or relationship structure?

    _____

    _____

    _____

5. If I am having a hard day, I would like my loved one to say this to me:

    _____

    _____

    _____

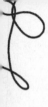

6. When I think about family building, I am:

    excited about... _____

    scared about... _____

    confused about... _____

After reflecting on these prompts, see if there are any values or priorities that consistently surface throughout your writing. Put another way: when you are rereading your answers, what matters most to you in your family building journey?

Four truths or values leading my journey:

1. _____

2. _____

3. _____

4. _____

2.

Barriers to Care and Obstacles to Equity

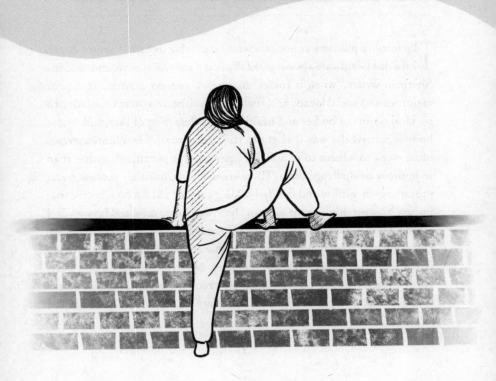

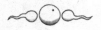

This part focuses on challenges in building your family in Canada, providing context and patterns in 2SLGBTQ+ peoples' access to equitable reproductive care. It is about the political and social landscape of our country's history and the presence, privileges, and oppressions that inform this access to care. It is not a precise prescriptive — it doesn't share what everyone will encounter in their own process. Read this part if you are interested in the background story that informs your own journey and the barriers that you and others might encounter on your path.

The fertility industry is not inherently equitable or just (Paynter 2022). Like our healthcare system generally, it is a *political* system, and as Zena Sharman writes, "when it comes to systems, context matters, as do our identities and social locations" (2021: 91). Healthcare systems are founded on ideal norms of bodies and health, who is deserving of care, and whose body functions the way it ought to (Sharman 2021). Healthcare systems often work to adhere to or solidify norms and expectations, rather than to improve or challenge them. There are many exclusionary processes and procedures in fertility and family-building care for 2SLGBTQ+ people that impact how we think about our care, how we pursue care, and how we feel asking questions about care. A lack of transparency in protocols, pricing, and regulations are major barriers to achieving equitable care in Canada (Ross et al., 2006; James-Abra et al. 2015; Marvel et al. 2016; Tam 2021; Kirubarajan et al. 2021b). And there are practical barriers, too, like forms that don't account for same-sex relationships or platonic co-parents, and digital health records that don't capture gender, sex, and sexual orientation beyond the categories of "male" and "female" (Antonio et al. 2022). It would be an error to decontextualize or dehistorize these barriers. It would be an oversimplification to see them as isolated challenges or easy fixes. We need to think through the complexities and layered ways that oppression operates, how the obstacles that oppress us might be part of a bigger story, and how the privileges some of us have access to are part of that narrative as well. I hope the next few sections can begin to situate your story, the individual experience of navigating a difficult system within much larger, longer, and more layered histories.

Throughout Part 2, I use a reproductive justice framework to explore fertility and family building for 2SLGBTQ+ people in Canada. The term *reproductive justice* was coined by Black leaders in Chicago in 1994. They recognized that white mainstream women's rights and activist movements did not engage and could not defend Black women's or other marginalized groups' rights (SisterSong 2023). At its foundations, reproductive justice is an intersectional movement, created by Black women, that brings together reproductive rights and social justice frameworks. Reproductive justice gives us language to speak about how rights, autonomy, power, and surveillance intersect and shape our current fertility care in Canada. It provides a lens for integrating decolonial, racial, disability, and class justice, among other intersectional experiences. Underlying the key concepts of reproductive justice is the reality that we cannot detach race, identity, community, and social context from experiences and outcomes of reproductive experience, sexual health, and fertility (Ross and Solinger 2017).

Our fertility journeys, our pregnancies, our labour, and our families do not exist in vacuums. They are tied together: How much access you have, how comfortable you feel advocating for your needs, how safe you feel questioning protocols, the ease with which you express your needs are all shaped by the historical and present ways people *like you* have been and are treated. Reproductive justice provides us with a framework for understanding how access to care, and expectations of oppression are inextricably tied to diverse histories of exclusion, sterilization, and birth evacuations for marginalized peoples in Canada (Choudhury 2016; Ross 2018; Smietana, Thompson, and Twine 2018). Reproductive justice shares two essential ideas for our family-building journeys: 1) access to comprehensive reproductive and sexual healthcare is a right; and 2) a right must apply equally, equitably, and accessibly to all people (Ross and Solinger 2017). It is a movement for abortion rights or the right to *not* have a child and a movement for the right to have a child and parent them with safety and dignity. People "should be able to have the number of children they want, when they want, in the way they want to have them" (Ross and Solinger 2017: 171).

Naming the barriers you might experience during this journey requires us to understand some of the foundational ways reproduction and families have been surveilled, managed, and controlled historically and currently. Accessible reproductive care includes economic access and ensuring available services, but it also means making reparations and reshaping the current healthcare system, so that there is both community leadership from those who have been historically and are currently oppressed as well as ongoing community consultations for how training, services, and care will best meet their needs. Access to fertility clinics and reproductive care is not neutral and cannot be detached from historical and current acts of discrimination and othering (Cranston-Reimer 2019).

With this historical context and theoretical framework in mind, the remainder of this part aims to unpack historical and ongoing barriers to care by situating current regulations within recent histories, exploring the impacts of medicalization on family building, considering the ongoing impacts of racism and settler colonialism on both intended families and donor availability, examining stigmatization and discrimination based on HIV status, and exploring how all of these factors compound to shape our expectations and anxieties around reproductive access. These challenges are not inevitable, and they are not universal. You may experience some of them or you might not experience any. *All journeys are different.* My goal is to help situate your interactions, experiences, and rights within a wider national project.

CONTEXT FOR CARE: HISTORY OF THE ASSISTED HUMAN REPRODUCTION ACT

Reproductive justice enables us to think critically about "wins" and understand how power operates to regulate experience even when we achieve better visibility or access to care through federal and provincial policies. Indeed, how we define family, make family, or at times conceal family are all products of dominant norms and ideologies. The history of 2SLGBTQ+ families does not begin with reproductive technologies — our families have always existed, in our histories of same-sex partnerships, chosen families, multi-parent families, undocumented and criminalized families, and co-parenting and platonic families. We exist across cultures, across geographies, across time. The history of this country is also the history of normalizing and "straightening" families: which families are seen as valued citizens, which people are seen as worthy of parentage, and which are refused the possibility of parenthood. This is because policies around family building are also tied to policies related to sterilization, privatized healthcare systems, and how reproductive technologies are marketed and consumed. While reproductive technologies are only one part of the story, they demonstrate how "the nation-state's intervention into reproduction is always already biopolitical" (Cranston-Reimer 2019: 67). A brief outline of the history of regulating reproductive technologies helps us connect the dots to see how the barriers that 2SLGBTQ+ people continue to experience today are a result of regulations and medicalization that purport to "protect" vulnerable populations but often fail to prioritize the needs they articulate.

In 1989, Brian Mulroney's government established the Royal Commission on New Reproductive Technologies to investigate "the ethical, legal, social, economic, and health implications" (Marvel 2016: 97) of new reproductive technologies and to develop recommendations and safeguards. While the Royal Commission is often applauded for seeking input provided from feminist movements in Canada when it was first established, the story of the feminist perspectives included and excluded is much more complex (Marvel 2016; Scala 2009). Where radical feminists who were a catalyst for the Commission saw assisted reproductive technologies (ART) as the commodification of "women's bodies," other feminists saw them as an opportunity for liberation and empowerment. Those who were against reproductive technologies called for control, regulations, and laws to ensure that people with eggs and a uterus were not sold or commodified for patriarchal interests. Led by medical geneticist and pediatrician Patricia Baird, the commissioners also included lesbian professor of religion Grace Marion Jantzen. However, the commissioners did not include representation from people of colour, Indigenous communities, members of the disability community, or heterosexual infertile couples (Marvel 2016).

Importantly, Marvel cautions us against celebrating and pinkwashing the inclusion of feminist and lesbian voices and instead argues that regulations, medicine, and law can be used to normalize family structures, even while incorporating "feminist voices aimed ostensibly at emancipation and liberation" (2016: 116). The writing of the report, which would be published in 1993, was fraught with disagreements and mistrust among researchers, commissioners, and analysts. Certain types of quantitative and medical-scientific research were privileged, while qualitative research was seen as advocating for "feminist issues" rather than providing impartial analysis. Once the commission report was released, it focused heavily on cost-effectiveness and new technologies rather than impact on communities. The researchers were not permitted to provide policy recommendations and were expected to provide "objective data" without advice (Scala 2009). Marvel notes that while the 1993 report may have used feminist language, many scholars and activists accused the report of appropriating feminist positions and ideas while decontextualizing and depoliticizing them. Indeed, "Diana Majury accused the report of taking a "Pollyanna approach to equality" wherein racism, sexism, oppression, and "lesbian hatred" are framed as matters of individual opinion rather than as systemic and institutionalized discrimination" (Marvel 2016: 108). Public health policy became a medium for protectionist and gatekeeping rhetoric that medicalized and criminalized some forms of family building by putting up new barriers to accessing sperm, eggs, and community-based services (like grassroots or self-insemination). While some of these are medically driven (testing for sexually transmitted illnesses and putting measures in place to prohibit exploitation are important steps in gender equity and healthcare), others were questionable even at the time they were recommended. For example, the assumption that donating eggs is *inherently* exploitative doesn't consider the impacts of *not* paying a donor or the possibilities of being coerced to donate through socio-emotional pressure (Cattapan 2013). Second, it strips people with eggs of their rights to make choices about their bodies or assumes that with monetary incentives they would be unable to make ethical choices in their own best interest (Cattapan 2013). Despite seemingly working to receive input from feminist communities, "the infertile heterosexual couple emerged as the exemplary service user of this new form of regulated, sanitized, economized, and engineered form of technological reproduction" (Marvel 2016: 109).

In 2004, eleven years after the 1993 report was published, Bill C-13, the Assisted Human Reproduction Act (AHRA), passed and became law in Canada. Bill C-13 prohibited some practices and enabled others. No human cloning, no selling sperm or eggs, no paying for surrogacy, and no sex selection were among the prohibitions. Altruistic surrogacy, donating eggs and sperm without compensation, and using human embryos and stem cells for research were permitted. The AHRA was critiqued for lacking clarity, clear regulations, or guidance on how to appropriately meet the regulations it laid out, and information continues to be updated to provide further detail on how the act should be regulated and enacted. For example, in 2020, changes were made to enable people to use known donors without having to wait for a six-month quarantine period, making it theoretically easier for clinics to meet the Health Canada regulations and testing requirements for working with known donors. While these changes came into effect in 2020, as of 2024 there are still many clinics that are not equipped to meet regulations to work with known donors. Additionally, in 2020, new guidance was also released to govern which expenses can be reimbursed to a surrogate and the requirements for reimbursement protocols. Though meant to help intended parents and clinics work within the parameters of the regulations, for many families the steps to meet requirements remain unclear. Early in the process, people are uncertain what their rights are, what costs to anticipate, the role of the surrogacy agency, and who to work with.

MEDICALIZATION AND PRIVATIZATION

One of the key factors that continues to disenfranchise 2SLGBTQ+ people on their family-building journeys is cost. Fees for donor gametes, the cost of procedures, expenses like medications quickly become prohibitive. Concerns about the relationship between ART access, economic disparities, and class equity date back to AHRA's origin story. Marvel notes that in early considerations of reproductive technologies, some feminists who spoke out against ART asserted that the costs of IVF and other interventions could be employed "as a mechanism to keep [ART] out of the grasp of anyone but white middle-class women, thereby ensuring the sterility of the disabled, non-white, and lower classes. There was seen to be real potential for a new eugenics movement" (2016: 93). Similarly, Alana Cattapan looks at how a two-tiered system has always been ingrained in ART in Canada, since "the Royal Commission's identification of certain technologies as 'experimental' worked to legitimate the exclusion of many ARTs from coverage under provincial health insurance programs, particularly in Ontario" (2013: 205–6).

The medicalization of family-building processes and the assumed necessity of intervention with prescription drugs, IVF, or additional testing is just one way in which cost quickly escalates. For 2SLGBTQ+ people who are trying to build their families, "infertility treatments" are often deemed the starting point, rather than a response to a need. The impact of medicalization is twofold: 1) 2SLGBTQ+ intended parents are immediately classified as unable to conceive, in need of healing, and indeed even unwell; and 2) the cost and necessity of extensive medical intervention are justified.

Infertility, according to the World Health Organization (2023b) is a disease "defined by the failure to achieve a pregnancy after 12 months or more of regular unprotected sexual intercourse." For a family that doesn't have access to sperm or eggs, equating their need for a donor with infertility can lead to medical and health interventions, testing that may not be necessary, medications that may not be warranted. This categorization is not incidental. As Marvel notes, when the AHRA was first established, it worked to label and reposition non-medical issues like accessing gametes as medicalized issues and illnesses, setting those without gametes readily available as societally aberrant. Marvel (2016: 114) writes: "The process of locating and diagnosing medical pathology requires that it be marked as deviance from a norm, affirming one set of bodies and conditions as 'healthy' and designating others as in need of treatment." The association between lack of access to gametes and a medical diagnosis not only medicalizes the process of family building but positions the queer family automatically as both deviant and "in need of healing." Patients who have been unable to achieve pregnancy are categorized as infertile. However, patients who require a donor because their bodies do not create sperm or eggs are not by default infertile. When faced with the desire to build a family we might feel compelled to listen to trusted medical advice on what is the "fastest" route to reach parentage. While there is nothing wrong with this option and it is valuable and valid for families to pursue, it is important that it is situated as a *choice* to allow families the autonomy to decide their first preferences.

Many 2SLGBTQ+ patients report frustration with a lack of consistency and transparency in billing and costs in their family-building journeys (Ross et al. 2006; Marshall 2021). While every province in Canada has a distinct funding structure for fertility treatment (or lack thereof), there is no centralized space for 2SLGBTQ+ people to learn about what funding is available for them or how long they must wait to receive it. The failure to provide transparent and clear information on wait times and costs is in part due to a lack of standardization and legislation. In Ontario, where provincial funding covers one round of IVF retrieval and subsequent transfers (excluding medication, donor gametes, and embryo testing), there is no standard method for prioritizing patients on a clinic's waitlist. Individual clinics are allotted funds to distribute among their patients, but there is no transparency around how this is done. As Michelle Tam (2021) notes, this has resulted in "a two-tiered system," where people with funds can privately access care quickly or choose to wait and utilize public funding when it is available. Policies pertaining to funding for IVF across provinces become even less clear when a family opts for reciprocal IVF (where one parent's eggs are retrieved and transferred into another parent's uterus), because there are no specific regulations on what this would look like and if both individuals can access funded cycles. Additionally, while IUIs are covered by some provincial healthcare plans, clinics may have additional fees that are not listed or shared with patients prior to their consultations, such as a "processing fee," which can range anywhere from $400 to $750 per cycle — in addition to medication costs. Because there is a lack of clarity and transparency in how funding is allotted for IUI in Ontario, parents who are initially told that their IUIs are covered may later be told the clinic has run out of funding.

Many individuals pursuing family building are initially unaware of the costs associated with assisted reproduction in Canada or how their province allocates funding to the treatments, if at all. Patients have noted that unanticipated fees, not covered by provincial healthcare, at times necessitated that they stop their fertility protocols entirely (Gregory et al. 2022). The costs of sperm processing, storage, or washing are all at the clinic's discretion and rarely mentioned in initial consultations with a clinic. As Michelle Tam (2021: 3) notes, "The majority of fertility clinics in Ontario are privatized with no overarching provincial legislation or standardization to govern the practice or fees associated," making it difficult to assess how funds are distributed within and across Canada, who has access to them, or even how to properly budget for your care. While Gregory et al. (2022) have noted improved care over the last two decades for 2SLGBTQ+ family building, participants in their study nonetheless continue to call for more transparency and clarity in potential costs, processes for obtaining gametes, and explicit guides for how to navigate the process.

At the time of writing this book in 2024, Alberta and Saskatchewan do not offer funding and reimbursement towards fertility treatments. Quebec has a medically assisted reproduction (MAR) program that offers eligible residents some funding for IVF, IUI, and fertility preservation. Newfoundland has a $5,000 reimbursement for IVF cycles (up to three cycles). New Brunswick residents can use a one-time grant of 50 percent of incurred costs for fertility treatments, up to $5,000 (but this only applies to those who have been diagnosed with fertility challenges). Manitoba and Nova Scotia offer a 40 percent tax credit on up to $20,000 for most fertility treatments and medications ($8,000 in credit a year). The Ontario Fertility Program provides funding to specific fertility clinics to cover the cost of treatments for residents, including unlimited IUIs and one round of IVF (excluding medications and some "elective" add-ons). In 2024, British Columbia announced that they would be introducing fertility funding in 2025 that will fund one round of IVF for both treatment and medication — although things like age, eligible clinics, and anticipated wait times and prioritization or triaging haven't yet been outlined. Currently, Fertility Matters Canada (fertilitymatters.ca) and Kin (joinkin.care) provide up-to-date information on provincial funding on their websites, including potential tax reimbursements and fertility coverage.

The impact of privatized, for-profit fertility care in Canada influences patient access and equity, as well as healthcare regulations. Vanessa Gruben (2020: 144) notes that fertility is "one of the few private for-profit health care sectors in Canada that is primarily paid for by private finance (private insurance and out-of-pocket payments) and delivered by for-profit facilities." The privatized structure of fertility care is troubling both because it creates undeniable class-based discrimination and barriers, and also because regulations for privatized clinics are not always externally standardized, relying primarily on self-regulation or clinical guidelines to shape their practices. With this internal regulation, Gruben (2020: 147) explains, "Patients have fewer options for bringing complaints about providers and facilities, and these processes offer less effective remedies; and data collection, which is a key tool for promoting patient safety, is less rigorous." Privatized care is therefore problematic because it impacts both quality of care and equitable access to services. Ultimately, Gruben looks at the fertility care model in Canada as a cautionary tale against a two-tiered medical system.

ONGOING OPPRESSIONS, WIDESPREAD IMPACTS

While there is very limited intersectional data on the experiences of 2SLGBTQ+ Indigenous, Black and racialized families pursuing fertility and family-building services (Tam 2021; Kirubarajan et al. 2021a; Twine and Smietana 2022), studies on broader populations of racialized and ethnic minorities in Canada demonstrate how race and ethnicity exacerbate the challenges associated with fertility and reproductive health (Gill et al. 2019; Kirubarajan et al. 2021a). Reproductive justice gives us language to think about how historical and current oppressions shape access even when services or funding might be made available for family building. As Sharlee Cranston-Reimer argues, histories of oppression — particularly those that are directly related to reproductive and sexual health — influence who accesses available services. When it comes to who utilizes funded fertility treatments, they are "still really accessible only for some and therefore ... fostering the building of a nation of those people" (Cranston-Reimer 2019: 72). In their 2021 study, Kirubarajan et al. note that racialized patients' mistrust in fertility providers and their fears that practitioners would hinder rather than support conception are ongoing impacts of the histories of forced sterilization and exper-imentation on enslaved and colonized peoples. Akuffo-Addo et al. (2023: 940) similarly write that "mistrust of medical advances among racialized populations continues to persist. The mistrust reflects the historical injustices and current systemic deficiencies experienced by racialized and marginalized populations."

Forced or coercive sterilization and aggressive assimilation policies are present in a not-so-distant past in Canada and continue to shape our healthcare system (Stote 2017). As Tam (2021: 2) notes, "Legislated and non-legislated coerced sterilizations were and are currently used as a form of mass birth control for Black, Indigenous, and people of colour, as well as LGBTQ2S+ people." Since the 1960s, Canada's birth evacuation policy — founded on settler-colonial obstetric violence that began in the 1800s — requires all Indigenous pregnant people living on rural and remote reserves to evacuate their home communities between thirty-six and thirty-eight weeks into their pregnancy and travel to urban centres prior to birth — often with no community members, family, or supports present (Cidro et al. 2020). This practice still occurs in parts of rural Canada today, stripping Indigenous people of their rights, bodily autonomy, and community care. Fertility care and reproductive technologies feel not only uninviting, but also dangerously controlled, managed, and surveilled for BIPOC 2SLGBTQ+ peoples and others who find themselves at the intersections and pluralities of marginalized identities.

The impact of these oppressions extends beyond intended parents and families to shape who feels most comfortable voluntarily participating in other reproductive processes like donating gametes or acting as a surrogate for altruistic purposes. For families who are racialized or Indigenous, looking for donors or surrogates with similar identities to their own is often challenging and limited (Marvel et al. 2016; Karpman et al. 2018; Daniels and Golden 2004). There is a level of trust and privilege necessary to act as a donor in Canada because, unlike in the US, gamete donors in Canada are not paid for their donations. Donors also must undergo a series of physical and mental health assessments, with frequent follow-up appointments over the course of six months to a year, necessitating the free time and flexibility to travel to a clinic and trust in the doctors, nurses, administrators, and staff to care for you. At the time of writing, only one Black donor is available on the Canadian Origin Sperm Bank and of the eighty-four Canadian-compliant donors on the American donor catalogue Fairfax Cryobank, only three Black donors are available. Abbie E. Goldberg (2022: 2) explains that "LBQ women who seek sperm donors of color, and particularly Black sperm donors, encounter a dearth of options from commercial sperm banks, whose donors tend to be disproportionately White." While there are many reasons this could be the case, mistrust in providers and the overwhelming whiteness that already exists in sperm banks influences who is seen as the right or most suitable and desirable donor. Daniels and Golden (2004) argue that current sperm bank operations reflect eugenic practices from the early twentieth century, selling and commodifying idealized notions of racial purity and perpetuating myths around what the most desirable human traits are.

Investigations into the lack of donor gametes available in Canadian-compliant banks from Indigenous and racialized populations must seriously consider how ongoing inequities influence the voluntary or altruistic decision to donate. When the state continually attempts to control and oppress marginalized peoples' reproductive experiences and bodies, there is often no safe or meaningfully consensual way for Indigenous and racialized peoples to donate gametes on their own terms with confidence in the system. The cascading impacts of a lack of sperm and eggs from particular communities, ethnicities, and identities influences intended parents and future families who are hoping to build families that "look like them" and have similar histories, experiences, and identities. Our lack of donor diversity is a symptom of a system that continues to discriminate against people of the global majority.

"RISKY BEHAVIOUR": PRESUMPTIONS OF HIV AND DONOR AVAILABILITY

In 1996 the Canadian Human Rights Act was updated to prohibit discrimination against anyone living with HIV or AIDS (and extending to anyone who is perceived or assumed to live with HIV and AIDS); in 2010 the American Society for Reproductive Medicine endorsed fertility services for HIV-positive people; and as of 2013, people with HIV with an undetectable viral load are permitted to use IVF to create their families. Despite all of these recognitions and promises of access, current donor protocols fail to make space adequately and equitably for HIV-positive people or men who have sex with men to donate gametes.

Until April 2024, regulations in Canada prohibited "a man who has had sex with a man" (or a person who produces semen who has sex with another person who produces semen) from donating to a sperm bank unless they had abstained from sexual intercourse for at least three months prior. This directive was based on historical assumptions so ingrained within our system that they failed to acknowledge medical advances, medications, or testing standards. From its inception in the 1990s, the Royal Commission had "laid the foundation for a system that assumed the HIV-positive status of gay donors and effectively shut down grassroots women's organizations aimed at supporting lesbians and single women" (Marvel 2016: 107). On April 19, 2024, news outlets shared that Health Canada would be amending the directive used for screening donors to remove the ban on men who have sex with men. Their communication stated: "After a review of the latest scientific evidence and feedback received from recent consultations, Health Canada is updating the donor screening criteria for sperm and ova donors to adopt a more inclusive screening approach…. The new inclusive approach will replace the current men who have sex with men screening questions with gender-neutral, sexual behaviour-based donor screening questions" (quoted in Zafar 2024). Health Canada's shift follows a similar 2022 amendment to permit men who have sex with men to donate blood.

Until recently, the laws and regulations about storing, washing, and treating sperm from people living with HIV have been unclear. In a recent 2020 update to the Safety of Sperm and Ova Regulations, parameters were clarified with more leniency provided in using sperm from an HIV-positive donor. However, one of the main problems is that new regulations fail to distinguish between detectable and undetectable viral loads in semen. Many clinics, surrogates, and intended parents are unaware that people with undetectable viral loads are unable to transmit the virus. As such, not all clinics are open or able to work with known donors, and of the clinics that are able to meet Health Canada regulations for known donors, not all of them are willing or able to work with those living with HIV. Ultimately, both the assumption that men who have sex with men *will* contract HIV and the refusal to account for the impact of antiretroviral drugs on HIV transmission demonstrate ongoing stigma and unfounded assumptions that equate an identity with inherent risk.

MINORITY STRESS THEORY AND CARE

The impact of historical oppressions, an imperative to undergo counselling, the prohibitive costs of using a fertility clinic, and ongoing homophobia and transphobia that exist in the country can all impact how we seek care, perceive care, and receive care. It is *stressful* and stress takes its toll both physically and emotionally. In the minority stress theory, there are two kinds of stressors we can experience that shape the emotional toll of starting a family: distal stressors and proximal stressors. Both are real and both can impact our mental and physical health. Distal stressors are external stressors like discrimination and rejection, and proximal stressors are internal stressors like internalized homophobia or simply *anticipating* discrimination. While someone might not have experienced stressors firsthand, the knowledge that others in their population have experienced these hardships in and of itself can have mental and physical impacts on individuals and families (Dorri and Russell 2022; Meyer 2015).

Minority stress causes psychological impacts — such as emotional dysregulation, social and interpersonal problems and depression, anxiety, and other adverse mental health outcomes — as well as neurobiological impacts that can mirror those found in people who experience PTSD and other stress-related disorders (Siegal et al. 2022). Micro- and macroaggressions such as incorrect names or pronouns, forms that do not provide options for diverse family structures, or the absence of images of similar families in print or digital materials can create a stress response that shapes our expectations and experiences in a medical environment. If we fill out a form at the doctor's office that assumes we are heterosexual, that doesn't include information or options for *our* families, then we might begin to feel excluded, a lack of representation, a sense of sadness, rage, or frustration. Before we even enter the physical clinic, we already have expectations of ostracism. Our stress levels are not a result of someone saying "you don't belong here" but of the ongoing explicit and implicit ways we are invited or excluded from a space. While not shaping all 2SLGBTQ+ family-building experiences, stressors like stigma and discrimination can regardless affect one's physical health (Minturn et al. 2021).

We also know that 2SLGBTQ+ minority stress is worse for some people than others. Having more social markers and experiences of marginalization amplifies the risk of oppression, violence, emotional distress, and even physical complications. Gato, Santos, and Fontaine (2017) looked at recent studies on minority stress in relation to queer and transgender parenting and found that experiences of minority stress are exacerbated for 2SLGBTQ+ people who are marginalized by their race and ethnicity. In thinking about the barriers to fertility and family building, mental health and proximal stressors shape our experiences from preconception through to parenthood. It's then more important to talk about and identify essential supports for healthcare, mental health, and community resources *now* before we are in the thick of our fertility journeys. Because we deserve good care. We deserve to be cared for. And we deserve community.

Studies have also shown that perinatal experiences affect the mental health and well-being of non-gestational parents, too, but they often have fewer resources and supports than birthing parents (Howat, Masterson, and Darwin 2023; Shenkman et al. 2022). There are some supports online for heterosexual fathers who are experiencing stress and mental health struggles related to pregnancy, loss, and parenting. However, there are significantly fewer supports for non-gestational 2SLGBTQ+ parents. The lack of these particular supports means that these parents are often in groups with cisgender heterosexual fathers, whose experiences rarely reflect their own.

PERFORMING OPTIMISM AND EVERYTHING IS FINE-ISM

Part of minority stress theory is understanding how inequities, anxieties, and oppressions shape how we "perform" in public spaces, what kinds of questions we feel comfortable sharing, and how open we are about challenges. 2SLGBTQ+ people end up feeling like they need to show up, smile on their faces, unfazed, unencumbered, and totally ready. They are afraid to show the normal cracks of wear and tear of fertility, parenting, mental health, because they fear there will be repercussions if they aren't just right. In their survey of studies on 2SLGBTQ+ perinatal mental health, Abirami Kirubarajan et al. (2022) found that all twenty-six studies reviewed identified multiple complex mental health challenges during the perinatal period for 2SLGBTQ+ childbearing individuals. Participants in the studies explained that there was frequently pressure to appear positive and optimistic. Two studies they looked at found that stigma and fear of discrimination resulted in a reluctance to pursue mental health diagnosis or support.

As Zena Sharman (2021: 47) explains, "too often, queer and trans people seeking to access health care are required to apply a veneer of 'normalcy' and 'respectability' to our lives and bodies to achieve a form of conditional acceptance inside a system that wasn't designed for us." In the world of fertility, this might mean not disclosing distress, mental health concerns, or trauma because of a fear of being seen as an inadequate or unfit parent.

Health Canada requires that those who use donor gametes complete *one* session with a therapist or counsellor. In theory, the idea is to prepare people for the experience of using a donor. But most frequently, this is an expensive check mark, where a therapist (often associated with a clinic) will meet once with a family and ask a series of questions that feel invasive, tedious, oppositional, or traumatic without any therapeutic relationship building or context (Gregory et al. 2022). While Health Canada does not require the therapist to be affiliated with a clinic or to have any specific designation that relates to fertility, clinics often have internal policies about who they will work with. The problem with this process is threefold: 1) To presuppose that some families or some family-building processes require more therapy or counselling than others is inequitable and unjust; 2) to control and manage who queer families receive counselling from implements an inequitable economic "queer tax" and deprioritizes the needs of the patient; and 3) a one-off session with someone you don't know, even the most well-meaning therapist, can feel like a test to see if you are fit to parent. Gregory et al. (2022: 3) note that some participants in their study felt that they needed to "give the 'right' answers to the questions posed by their counselor, for fear of 'failing the test' and being denied access to services … important questions that may feel neutral for the heterosexual patient population may elicit unintended consequences with lesbian patients." Expecting someone to be completely forthright with a stranger about their questions, fears, or anxieties about donor conception is unrealistic and unfair. As Sharman (2021: 48) continues, "Our health system often demands queer and trans people take the care we are given without complaint, even if it is violent, inadequate, or just plain wrong, often at great personal and/or financial cost." 2SLGBTQ+ people may feel they need to perform normativity, lie about their family structure or co-parenting arrangement, or conceal disabilities in order to access care.

Whose Policies Are They, Anyway?

Advocating for our needs necessitates that we understand our options. If a clinic is demanding costly out-of-pocket tests be performed, if they will only allow you to complete a mandated counselling session with their counsellors rather than someone of your choosing, or if they are requiring medications, protocols, or interventions that you are unsure about, ask who is making these requirements and if they are provincially or federally mandated or simply policies of the clinic. As someone trying to build your family, it is important to know that it is okay to ask questions, to bring a partner or support person with you to ask questions, or to speak with a clinic manager to determine what options are within your control and what are currently necessary according to federal or provincial mandates.

STRATEGIES FOR SYSTEMIC SHIFTS

My goal is not to point fingers at any one clinic. I have never met a doctor or a nurse who has said "I want to make my patient's life hard today," "I don't believe these people should be parents," or "I don't believe in 2SLGBTQ+ rights." I truly believe healthcare providers by and large have good intentions. But intentions do not preclude or excuse negative impacts, oppression, or discrimination against 2SLGBTQ+ patients. There is a fundamental systemic problem at the foundation of our fertility care, and the shifts that need to happen are beyond any one clinic. Among many other political and social changes to our system, we need:

♦ **Education and curriculum requirements.** Current curricula for health practitioners treat 2SLGBTQ+ care as supplementary, an afterthought, a continuing education seminar. Significant research has indicated the need for specific 2SLGBTQ+ training and education to improve health outcomes and experiences. Korpaisarn and Safer (2018) argue that a lack of gender-affirming and transgender-specific education among healthcare providers is a significant barrier for transgender patients and recommend integrating appropriate content to improve practitioners' proficiency in this area; Schreiber et al. (2021) affirm the need for integrated and standardized medical education for 2SLGBTQ+ curricula to better support patients, improve health outcomes, and improve provider competence; Lee et al. (2021) examine how targeted trainings and increased provider competence can improve the poorer health outcomes for 2SLGBTQ+ patients in comparison to age-matched cisgender/heterosexual peers; Nina et al. (2022) consider the need for guidelines and approaches to oncofertility for young adults who are sexual and gender minorities; and Gisondi and Bigham (2021) note that the gap in competence and population-specific knowledge for 2SLGBTQ+ healthcare is a "failure of medical education." We need a major shift in medical curricula to integrate 2SLGBTQ+ and gender-affirming care in every aspect of reproductive and fertility education. We are more than the services we seek, and the complexity of our identities, families, and relations is what makes us so beautiful.

+ **Economic equality and equitable funding.** Fertility care is a class issue. People with more access to funds and greater economic privilege can access more timely intervention, options for testing and protocols, and easier travel to clinics. Indeed, the main entry point of care is determined by class, making fertility care a kind of population control. Public funding for fertility care is essential to ensure that all people throughout the country are able to access their right to create the family they choose. Economic equity is intersectional: access to leisure time, to paid leave, to daycare, and to medications impacts access to services for intended parents, donors, and surrogates. In addition to public funding, we also need more transparency around costs and fees. Clinics should be required to provide up-to-date information to patients, including on administrative fees, procedural fees, and the range of costs for medications.

+ **Policy and regulatory amendments.** In our current system, policy intervention and regulations are a double-edged sword. We need to be included in regulations, in medical policies, and in healthcare systems, because sometimes we need or want medical intervention in our family-building care. But we also

know that regulations, medicalization, and criminal-
ization can mandate and enforce state surveillance
and control. These measures may at times support
our family building and at times hinder it. We need consistent
and ongoing consultation with diverse community members,
with participation in drafting recommendations and imple-
menting changes.

we're here, we're queer!

+ **Transparency in protocols and rights.** Clinics should provide
intended parents with access to plain-language reports on their
options for methods of conceiving, the federal and provincial
requirements, and where they can go if their needs are not being
met or they experience discrimination. Simple overviews that
cater to 2SLGBTQ+ people can make a world of difference in
ensuring autonomy, control, and consent from intended parents,
surrogates, and donors.

Because we might be waiting on major (and minor) shifts for a
long time, we also need each other. We need to learn to advocate for
ourselves and to build our support teams for when we cannot do so.
We need to talk about the consequences of silence and the ongoing
impact of systemic oppression. We need to protect our bodies as we
prepare for pregnancy or family building, and we need to have our
experiences and hardships acknowledged. On top of all of these practical shifts and systemic changes, we also need to get comfortable with
complexity and the simultaneous recognition of how far we have come
and how much further we have to go. We can celebrate personal victo-
ries, feel excited to receive funding, acknowledge newfound visibility,
and applaud advocacy wins. At the same time, we can mourn losses,
feel the weight of silenced or erased voices, challenge how disability,
race, fatness, neurodivergence, gender diversity, and other markers

of "difference" still make family building less feasible for many, and rage at a system that can make us feel small, invalid, or unseen. *All* of this can be true at the same time. Your story is part of a history of advocacy, activism, and reproductive justice movements that have fought for change, access, and visibility. There are still incredible challenges and fights to be won. There is still so much to do.

3.

Building Community and Strategies for Collective Care

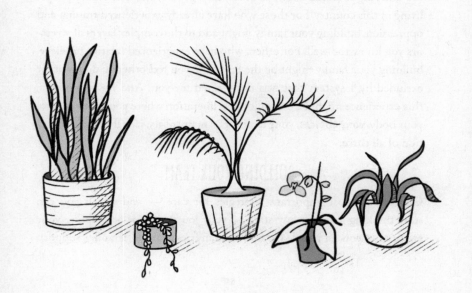

This part is about community and collectivity; it is about caring for yourself and for each other; it is about learning how to identify your choices, take agency, and problem solve when your plan goes off course. Read this part if you are looking to navigate hard conversations and make big choices or if it looks like your choices may not be possible. These pages are all about your team, building community, and recognizing resources. We need to strategize our care when it is not a given.

While there are books that can prepare you for the first steps of starting a family, there are few that acknowledge the emotional and physical toll of trying to start a family as queer, transgender, and non-binary people living in this country. For those who have already experienced trauma and oppression, building your family might add to the complex layers of stressors you know too well. For others who have experienced relative privilege, building your family might be the first time you feel othered, different, or excluded by a system that was not created for you. And for still others, this experience might be one of joy and liberation where you get to control your body, your choices, your family. For many of us, it will be a combination of all three.

BUILDING YOUR TEAM

One of the most important strategies for care — and which you can start thinking about at any stage of your journey — is assembling your team: a network of people (or non-human friends) who can offer support, care, resources, and information at the beginning of this journey and into parenthood and aging. Each of our teams looks different and each of our teams will necessarily change. Strategies for care are not solely about understanding the process of healthcare and medicine or identifying the obstacles and challenges that might make it hard for you to access your care; it is also crucial to understand how you fit in the lineages of queer, transgender, and non-binary families who have laboured, fought, and carved out spaces for our rights, existence, and love and who continue to do so. Queer and transgender communities are multiple and overlapping, different, and disparate. There is no single 2SLGBTQ+ community and there is no single way to make a family.

In the lines below, list your own "team members" to remind yourself of the community supports, resources, people, and things you have in your corner, when things get hard.

Chosen family. Sometimes our family — the ones who feel close or understand us — are blood kin, the people to whom we are biologically linked. Sometimes our family are the tightly knit friendships that are more than friendships. The people who will be there for us no matter how seldom we talk. Sometimes our families are changing: we allow our relationships to ebb and flow, with different people filling different needs, each of us playing a different, shifting role in each other's lives.

_____

_____

_____

Friends. Our team is also composed of friendships, old and young, human and non-human. Think of the friends that construct your support network. Check in with them about their desire and ability to support you in your journey of trying to build your family and in your parenting years ahead. Try not to make assumptions about what care looks like to friends or family. We all have different ideas of support, showing up, and providing care. Be honest about your expectations of friendships and how they might change while preparing for (and then after) a little human arrives.

_____

_____

_____

Mental health support. Now is the time to think about how your mental health might be impacted by trying to build your family, the processes of pregnancy, surrogacy, or non-gestational pregnancy, and postpartum periods. Our team members can be formal mental health practitioners, psychiatrists, social workers, therapists, and they can also be informal mental health supports: furry family members and pets, social media accounts and influencers, podcasts, or literature, fidget toys, or coping mechanisms. Our team isn't just people. Our team are the objects, beings, resources that make us feel a sense of community. Think about what mental health supports look like to you and make a list or mind map of supports that might be useful as you move through this process.

_____

_____

_____

Doctors and other healthcare providers. Your healthcare team might comprise a family doctor, a walk-in clinic, fertility nurses, or reproductive endocrinologists (REIs), or it might involve naturopathic doctors or acupuncturists, massage therapists, or other care practitioners. When you are building your family, there may be new physical experiences, side effects, or symptoms that you aren't familiar with. Telehealth or urgent care phone numbers can be useful to have on hand on this journey. Each province and territory in Canada offers telehealth frameworks that work with their provincial health plans and in a national context; calling 8-1-1 can give you access to free 24/7 registered nurses. (Residents of Manitoba can call 204-788-8200 to access this service.) Though these aren't always perfect resources, they can be useful if you have immediate non-emergency questions.

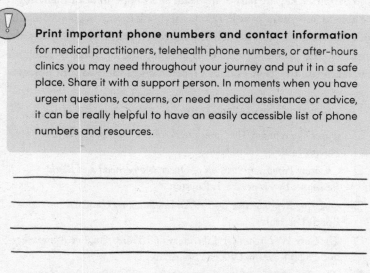

Print important phone numbers and contact information for medical practitioners, telehealth phone numbers, or after-hours clinics you may need throughout your journey and put it in a safe place. Share it with a support person. In moments when you have urgent questions, concerns, or need medical assistance or advice, it can be really helpful to have an easily accessible list of phone numbers and resources.

Books and authors. Building your team is also about building your library. The authors, activists, storytellers, and birth workers who support us in planning and building our families are invaluable parts of our team. We can bring their voices and words into our experience like a firm hand to hold — people to walk alongside us and give us words of encouragement, validation, an understanding of the obstacles and barriers we face as 2SLGBTQ+ people. Who is in your library?

_____

_____

_____

I wrote this book in conversation with other books, authors, experts, and parents. They are part of my team and I hope some of them might be able to join yours as well. I hope this book is read in good company and that we may speak to each other through your own reflections and insights. The people who have inspired me and continue to teach me can teach you too! Some books I recommend adding to your library:

- ☐ *Baby Making for Everybody: Family Building and Fertility for LGBTQ+ and Solo Parents* by Ray Rachlin and Marea Goodman

- ☐ *Queer Conception: The Complete Fertility Guide for Queer and Trans Parents-to-Be* by Liam Kali

- ☐ *Choosing Family: A Memoir of Queer Motherhood and Black Resistance* by Francesca T. Royster

- ☐ *Queering Reproductive Justice: An Invitation* by Candace Bond-Theriault

- ☐ *The Care We Dream Of: Liberatory and Transformative Approaches to LGBTQ+ Health* by Zena Sharman

- ☐ *And Baby Makes More: Known Donors, Queer Parents, and Our Unexpected Families* by Chloe Brushwood Rose and Susan Goldberg

- ☐ *Reproductive Losses: Challenges to LGBTQ Family-Making (Gender and Sexualities in Psychology)* by Christa Craven

- [ ] *Taking Charge of Your Fertility: The Definitive Guide to Natural Birth Control, Pregnancy Achievement, and Reproductive Health* by Toni Weschler (Note: This book contains gendered language and is not geared towards 2SLGBTQ+ communities. I am adding it to the list because it offers comprehensive guidance on cycle charting and understanding ovulation and menstrual cycles.)

And because the journey is only just beginning:

- [ ] *Essential Labor: Mothering as Social Change* by Angela Garbes
- [ ] *Raising Antiracist Children* by Britt Hawthorne
- [ ] *Good Inside: A Guide to Becoming the Parent You Want to Be* by Becky Kennedy

Elders and ancestors. Our identities are shaped by our chosen families and intimate kin, by the elders we've met and those of which we have no direct memory, along with the resistance of those who have fought for our practices, rituals, beliefs, and relationships to continue. Take a moment to think about the vast lineages of peoples, communities, families, non-human kin, friends, elders and ancestors who are part of your journey. What does your team look like and who can you reach out to if you need support?

Our team isn't just made up of the people you can call on the phone for help (though they are important!); it is also about the people whose stories and histories give us strength and empower us to advocate for our needs.

_____

_____

_____

_____

DIGGING ROOTS AND GROWING BRANCHES: A FOREST OF QUEER KINSHIP

We use trees to represent family lineages, ancestries, and connections. I invite you to think beyond the names and labels of the traditional "family tree" and instead to expand your understanding to build your networks through the metaphor. Get some pencil crayons and let's have some fun.

Colour in the roots. Think about what is at your foundation. Write the names of the people you are growing from, those who continue to ground you. It might be a blood ancestor, it might be someone you know well, it might be chosen family, or someone you have never met.

Colour in the branches. Limbs allow you to reach. They might be people who help you extend. They might be parents, siblings, cousins, friends. They might be values or experiences.

Colour in your leaves. The leaves can change colour, grow, create awe, and represent change. What are the things or people who add glitter and beauty to this step of your journey, whose roles can change, or presence is temporary?

Colour in your trunk. A trunk is you, your partner(s), your family. This is your centre, and it is also your home. A strength. A pillar. Fill in the trunk with words and images that depict your hopes and your fears, that make you feel home. You are complicated and beautiful, and your family is connected and strong.

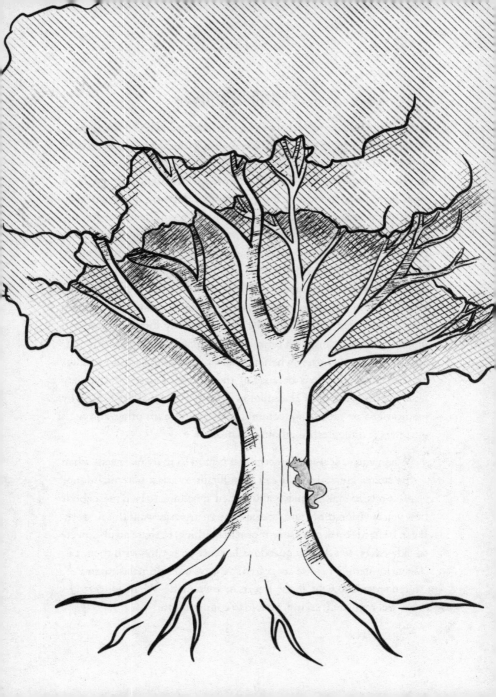

COMMUNICATION

A lot of the books and websites you may read will tell you the steps to IUIs, what to expect from IVF, how to deal with the stress and anxiety, and even how you can ask someone to be your donor. These are all incredibly important steps and knowledge. Suddenly, we go from wanting to be a parent to being a therapist, a doctor, a nurse, a negotiator, and a researcher. We are propelled into a wild world of fertility and relationship building. And sometimes we forget, speeding along that road, about the importance (and the need) for communication. Communicating to your partner(s) or support system, communicating with your doctors or nurses (and advocating further if you don't feel heard), communicating with potential donors, communicating with family about our choices, and the one we usually forget or diminish most: communicating with ourselves. There are many times throughout the perinatal journey when it is hard to communicate our feelings or needs. Whether it is because of the increased stress and anxiety from coping with all of the unknowns or hormonal shifts caused by medications or pregnancy, communicating with each other and with ourselves is difficult throughout this process.

When you're scared. Sometimes it is hard to share our needs when the stakes are so high. It can be difficult to ask a potential donor questions, to make requests about their timelines, to be honest about how you envision the future, because you so urgently want this to work. It can be hard to ask a nurse to repeat something, to share an unexpected side effect, to ask new questions because your time with them can feel *so* limited. When we are scared, we leave our optimal state and often enter into fight, flight, freeze, or fawn mode. We no longer feel regulated, secure, or able to communicate.

fight

flight

fawn

freeze

When you're angry. When we are angry, when we feel rushed, when we feel out of control, it is often because of a communication barrier: we aren't feeling heard, and we aren't hearing the other person. Communication requires us to press *pause* so we can listen. And we usually don't do this as well as we think we might. We often have fears, anxiety, past traumas, and past circumstances that can make it hard for us to listen to intention rather than assumption, and this is especially true when we aren't hearing ourselves.

When you're feeling vulnerable. It can be easier to *not* hear ourselves, because hearing ourselves can be vulnerable and hearing our fears can be scary. Communication requires us to make space for our feelings, understanding what sets us off, when we shut down, and the barriers for expressing our needs. We teach children to count to ten and take a deep breath when they feel rage or overwhelm, because we know that this whole-body experience can make it hard to control our impulses, stay calm, and be in the moment. But sometimes as we grow older, we forget how much those tools apply. And learning how to take a breath, how to count to ten, how to set your own boundaries, are all tools that you not only need right now but will also need to model and share with your future family.

Understanding communication barriers through dysregulation. We face major barriers when we try to communicate while in a dysregulated, emotional state. The stress of fertility and family building can trigger a lot of emotions, discomfort, and fears. It is essential that we focus on how that impacts our communication, so that we can be there for each other, share our needs, and hear others' needs.

In his book, *The Developing Mind* (1999), Dan Siegel suggests that we all have a range of intensities of emotions that we are able to experience, process, and integrate with relative ease or comfort. He calls this our *window of tolerance*. When we are in our "window" we have control over our emotions, communications, and behaviours. We have smooth sailing! When we are triggered, we move outside of our window of tolerance and feel less in control. We become either *hypo-aroused* or *hyper-aroused*. Survival modes kick into gear, our rational thinking goes out the window, and our emotions and reactions are dominated by survival instincts (fight, flight, freeze, or fawn). How wide our window is and what moves us into these different states is different for everyone. For some of us it is quite narrow, and small things can make us feel out of control. For others, our windows are wide, it takes more for us to feel dysregulated. The width of our window can be a result of our experiences, trauma, relationships, and coping mechanisms. This is important: Your window width is not anything you did wrong or to be ashamed of. And understanding your triggers and barriers can help you understand why you are struggling to communicate and begin to identify what you need in order to get back to a more optimal state.

When stressors take us above our window, we may feel anxiety, panic, anger, or disassociation. In this state of hyper-arousal, we might feel aggressive or defensive, have heightened emotional reactivity, or feel like we just can't calm down. With this flood of intense emotions, we may be less able to engage in problem solving and communications. If our arousal level goes below our window of tolerance, we might shut down, feel numb, feel disconnected. Hypo-arousal can cause decreased sensitivity to stimuli, less awareness of our surroundings, and difficulty concentrating. In this state it can be hard to mobilize energy, motivation, or have meaningful conversations.

We need to be able to name and acknowledge when we are outside of our optimal state, so that we can opt out of hard conversations and make space for strategies to return to our window of tolerance. There are many different kinds of strategies for getting back in our optimal zone; I already discussed one (don't underestimate the impact of taking really good, deep breaths!).

There are other techniques that work well for many people. Talk with a mental health provider when trying to figure out techniques that work best for you. The following are some options:

+ **Square or "4 x 4" breathing.** In this style of breathing, you begin by breathing out, releasing air from your lungs. Now, breathe in slowly through your nose, counting to four in your head. Hold your breath for a four-count. Now exhale for another four counts. Hold for four, then inhale again, repeating the process. You can do these three or four times (inhale for four, hold for four, exhale for four, hold for four). You can do this throughout the day to give yourself practice, so that in moments of overwhelm or triggers, the tool is more easily accessible to you.

+ **Grounding yourself.** Grounding exercises can help you to tap into physical sensations (touch, sight, sound, taste) and anchor yourself in the present moment. If you are experiencing overwhelm, this can be as simple as sitting in a chair, feet on the ground, and naming the objects that you see. Tuning into the physical can help you to regulate in the moment.

+ **Reconnecting with your body.** Somatic experiencing teaches us that we can work with our nervous system and release tension by discharging physical energy in activities like leaning or pushing into a physical wall. This allows your body to release stress and can help to reregulate your system. Stand near a wall and plant your hands against it. Grounding your feet on the floor, take a deep inhale and as you exhale firmly push against the wall, with your arms fully extended. Acknowledge all of the muscles working to create this force, from your legs to your arms, to your back, and to your glutes. Feel the weight of your body in the balls of your feet. Increase or decrease the strength of your push, in whatever way feels right for you. Repeat for as long as feels right for your body.

+ **Mindfulness and meditations.** Exercises and apps that help you to navigate meditation can be helpful for getting back into your window. Things like colouring, knitting, or even playing solitaire can be part of a mindfulness and meditation practice too!

Ultimately, our goal is widening our window of tolerance (but that is a whole other book and specialty!). The objective of this part is really to get you thinking about how our emotional state can impact our communication practices and how important our communication practices are to our family-building journeys. This is really just the beginning of learning about how you communicate, how you listen, and how you have hard conversations, because there will be many in your reproductive journey and even more as you navigate parenting.

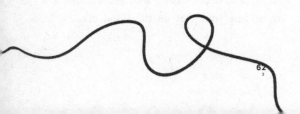

BOUNDARIES AND FAMILY
by Anna Balagtas

Anna Balagtas brings her experience as a non-binary birth worker, mentor, educator, community leader, and reproductive justice advocate to shape doula access, education, and supports and address gaps in knowledge, programming, and mentorship. Here, she shares her insights on and deep understanding of the tough conversations 2SLGBTQ+ people often need to have in the early stages of their journey.

Queering Conception When Your Relatives Are Rooted in Cis-hetero-monogamy

This section is written for queer families who are not understood by family members who hold traditional colonial, monogamous cis-heterosexual values. It addresses ways of setting boundaries and practising self-care while you're in your queer TTC journey that may help you protect your capacities should homophobia, transphobia, and any other queerphobias present within your relationships.

In this section, "family" refers to blood family relatives. "Chosen family" are the people you choose to bring into your circle, your space, your heart, or your home. Sometimes these relations overlap and sometimes they do not. I use the terms distinctly here to differentiate the two — each of us can find our place (and our family members' places) somewhere in the blurry lines within and between these terms.

What Does Queering TTC Look Like?

Let's first begin by naming what queering up the TTC journey may look like. If you identify as queer, anything you do is inherently queer, as is your experience of this process. Your queerness is valid even if you are in a monogamous cis-heterosexual relationship. Below, I have listed a few ways of queering conception that may leave room for curiosity from members of your family (even if this curiosity is not welcomed). This is only a short list of examples, but I hope parts of you are reflected in what is written. Regardless of who you are and your positions, I see you. I care for you. I support you. I love you.

+ Conceiving on your own

+ Conceiving with a partner

+ Conceiving with multiple partners

+ Conceiving with a partner while unmarried

+ Conceiving with multiple partners while unmarried

+ Conceiving with multiple partners while married

+ Conceiving simultaneously with a partner

+ Conceiving simultaneously with partners

+ Conceiving with a surrogate

+ Conceiving within a community or commune

+ Conceiving with chosen family

There are many ways to conceive that leave room for questions from folks who are approaching it with a cis-hetero-monogamous lens. Many times, traditionally minded family members will assume that only folks who are in cis-heterosexual, married relationships should have children together — and this is so far from the truth.

What to Do with "Family Disapproval"?

Most often a family's disapproval of queer fertility comes from family members not understanding the structure of your queerness, queer relationships, and queer family building. Having said this, it is *not* your responsibility to educate your family when you have no capacity. It's difficult enough to have your identity and positionality questioned but coupling that with having to explain the *validity* of your existence and choices can be too much.

In moments where you may find yourself needing to explain the validity of your queerness and family building, it's important to remember that asking your family members to outsource their learning where it doesn't include you being their teacher is a perfectly reasonable boundary and a means of protecting your capacity. Your response to their request to teach them can sound something like:

> Thank you for wanting to learn more about my queer family dynamics — it makes me feel really held and seen. I'm excited that you're actively wanting to educate yourself on the things that you know are important to me, but I don't have the capacity to teach you myself. I do know of some great resources that can get you started, though! I know it's easier if you were to learn from me directly, but having to constantly teach folks about my identities, values, and how to respect them starts to become exhausting and I want to make sure I'm protecting my capacities. Thank you for understanding!

There are many folks who do the active work of educating people on queerness and family building, and you can point your family to these resources rather than taking on the potentially exhaustive labour of explaining it yourself.

Communicating Your Boundaries

Communicating your boundaries can look many ways. If it's within your capacity, you can have an in-person chat with your family members and tell them how you are feeling and what you need from them or what you will no longer accept from them. If it's easier for you, write out your boundaries on paper or on your notes app and read them directly so you don't miss one. You can also communicate your boundaries by way of text, a call, or over email. If in-person is not within your capacities, perhaps it's best to do it from the comfort of your home.

Communicating your boundaries might mean saying...

+ "It makes me uncomfortable when you question the ways I want to conceive/build my family because it makes me feel like you're invalidating my choices. Please stop questioning my decisions; otherwise I'll opt for not sharing them with you any longer."

+ "If you'd like to ask me about my family planning, it will feel best for me to talk by _____" [texting, calling, seeing each other in person — choose whatever means of communicating feels best for you!].

Another way you could communicate your boundaries is by way of a person you trust — perhaps your partner, a chosen family member, or an understanding blood family member can name your boundaries for you. As long as your needs and boundaries are articulated, there is no wrong way of communicating.

You absolutely don't need to explain yourself when it comes to your boundaries. If you don't feel like explaining why you chose to enforce the boundaries you have, you don't need to. You can explain as little or as much of why you're setting boundaries, but in general — you don't owe anyone a reason.

What Is Your Hard Stop?

Think of your *hard stop*. A hard stop is a point at which you no longer have capacity for engaging with particular family members. When do you think a *hard stop* may need to be called? What are actions or dynamics we can put into place so we don't get to this point?

I want to remind you that calling a hard stop on family doesn't mean you no longer love and respect your family member(s) — actually, it shows just how much you love them by putting in place a system where your capacities are protected, your being is respected, and your relationships with each other can still be nurtured — even if it has to be from afar.

Practical Strategies for Self-Care

Take a deep breath. These reflections may be a hard read for some of you! In honouring this, I'd invite you to think of some ways you can nurture yourself at this time and in the moments involving your family members where you may need to step away for self-care. Below is a quick list to get you started, but stay curious with yourself and add to or remove from this list in ways that feel best for you.

- Set and name your boundaries
- Journal, make art, record voice notes: explore everything that is on your mind without editing your thoughts — just keep writing, talking, making art without judgment
- Talk out your feelings with partner(s), chosen family, a counsellor, or trusted members of your community
- Find ways to validate your queerness and your queer family building by joining groups, collectives, forums filled with folks who are moving through similar experiences as you

- Chat with queer families and find community with them
- Take time where you *don't* talk about queer TTC and families
- When we are dealing with stress, we are in an activated state — explore what you need in a state of activation to settle your nervous system
- Meditate, find out what your body needs

Remember, you are a unique and authentic person and your self-care must reflect that. Only you will know what you want and need in the moment and though I've listed some examples of things you could do, ultimately whatever you choose as self-care is entirely valuable.

ACTIVITY

• • •

PERSONAL REFLECTIONS

What are your soft boundaries? These are the boundaries you are flexible with — meaning you may find it annoying when they are crossed but it does not ultimately send you spiralling.

_____

_____

_____

What are your hard boundaries? What are boundaries you absolutely will not tolerate being crossed?

_____

_____

_____

What measures do you have in place to protect your energy? This could look like creating sanctuary spaces in your home, rituals, debriefing with a counsellor, etc.

_____

_____

_____

_____

If you choose to educate your family members and provide them with resources, who are the people you will point them to so they may further their learning (websites, organizations, support people)?

_____

_____

_____

_____

Aside from yourself, who can support you in enforcing your boundaries?

_____

_____

_____

_____

What are your partner(s)' relationships to other family members (if applicable)?

_____

_____

_____

_____

A Means for Compromise

After all of this talk of creating soft boundaries, hard boundaries, and hard stops within our relationships with our family members, I think it's important to end on a note of compromise.

Perhaps compromise is something that you can implement in your relationships now, or perhaps this is something that you will revisit in the future. A compromise with your family regarding your queer conception journey can look like a lot of different things. A compromise might look like having your family involved, without being overly involved — their presence is not black and white, and limits can be fluid and shift. You can use specific tools for communication and create boundaries on how much time spent is together. You deserve your space and don't owe anyone an explanation as to why you may choose to keep some folks at bay. You are allowed to give them some updates about a pregnancy or family-building journey but refuse to engage with unwanted questions and comments regarding the process of conception: "That's not something we are sharing."

Compromise can also look like queering traditions. Instead of a gender reveal party where the premise revolves around binary gendering, have a party where you celebrate the spectrum of genders (or no gender). This can also be a big learning moment for family members who don't have a concept of genders outside the binary. Celebrations can be times to honour your family without entertaining or answering any questions about your family-building journey: "Today we aren't talking about that. We are celebrating our family."

Recommended Reading:

+ *Set Boundaries, Find Peace* by Nedra Glover Tawaab

COMPASSIONATE, CONSCIOUS, COLLECTIVE CARE: ENGAGING THE C3 MODEL

A Conversation with Gabrielle Griffith

> *In this conversation, Gabrielle Griffith (they/them) shares their tools for community care and why we need to think about community building, mental health, and postpartum support at the early stages of family building. Gab is a birth worker, an activist, and a leader in 2SLGBTQ+ fertility, pregnancy, and postpartum support. They have contributed to a number of initiatives supporting 2SLGBTQ+ families, including being program coordinator for Seed and Sprout at Birth Mark. C3 Care is a care model they developed for internal reflection, identifying community supports, and conversations about accountability and consent to have with your friends, chosen family, and support networks. The strategies and tools discussed here help you to think about how to set up the necessary care and resources for your perinatal journey, from preconception to postpartum community and collective care.*

Laine Halpern Zisman: This conversation is really an opportunity to reflect on the work that you do to support intended parents and new parents and what drives you to do it. Do you want to start by introducing yourself?

Gabrielle Griffith: My name is Gabrielle Griffith. I use they/them pronouns. I am a parent, doula, community organizer, and program coordinator of Seed and Sprout at Birth Mark Support, organizing 2SLGBTQ+ family programming. In this season of my life, I'm looking for intentional ways to bridge the gaps in 2SLGBTQ+ communities, particularly for people with little humans or those looking to care for little humans. And to find ways to bring each other together and support one another.

LHZ: What made you want to do this work with 2SLGBTQ+ communities?

GG: It was my own pregnancy experience. I don't think that I would be where I am or who I am today had I not been blessed with an unexpected pregnancy. I made the decision to keep my kiddo at that point in time. Through my pregnancy I just became a lot more comfortable with myself and my body. I didn't come out as queer until I was eight months pregnant and found ways to become more comfortable with myself and take up more space within the community.

I had a very lonely, very sad postpartum experience and very much remember being in the depths of that, knowing that this isn't what it's supposed to be like. But also not having any insight on how to make things different. Learning about doula work and community, I realized how different my birth and postpartum would have been with those supports. From there, through all of the different readings I did and my own lived experience, I developed the care model that we're going to talk about today. I call it C3 Care: Conscious, Compassionate, Collective Community Care.

LHZ: Thank you so much for sharing that and being so open and vulnerable about your postpartum experiences. I feel like so many people experience this loneliness and don't know where to go or how to access resources. When you're trying to start your family, in these initial stages, there aren't a lot of people who are talking about postpartum depression or anxiety, and it can hit a lot of people by surprise.

GG: It's funny because in the early stages of family building, we are so focused on material and tangible things — things that you can touch— finding sperm or eggs or a surrogate, preparing for a crib, buying the right blankets and clothes and diapers and wipes, which are all important in their own way. But we aren't thinking intentionally about *our* needs or how we envision community.

I remember I went through a blogging phase, and I wrote this blog about being a new mom and the experience of no one around me asking me, "How are *you*?" Like, how are you *really* doing? How does it feel to be a mother? And honestly, it felt awful. I think the reason that people hesitate to talk about postpartum experiences in advance is because if we really got to the nitty gritty of the duality of parenting (how fantastic it is, but also how exhausting it is) I think it might turn some people away from the idea of it or might make people second guess their capacity to do it.

Sometimes we are surrounded by people but we feel alone, either because we haven't talked about what care looks like to us or what we might need or be able to do. There is such a big gap in the conversation when we're discussing postpartum care: you have all these amazing supports and this plan for *the baby*, but what are you going to do for yourself?

LHZ: So, C3 Care is a care model that tries to help people intentionally think through that. How did that come about?

GG: When I was in my postpartum period the only other person in my life at that point in time, who was supporting me with my child, was his father. And that was great and helpful in the sense that I would get days off to myself, but I realized that wasn't enough and that time off wasn't actually restorative for me. I was missing community for myself. My kiddo was very well taken care of, and I was not very well taken care of.

C3 Care comes from my lived experience of that. From journals, lots of trial and error of trying to find people, identifying needs and resources, and therapy sessions. It was a time for me to find ways to work through the blockages and negative self-thoughts that I was experiencing, and then sharing this information with the people around me. I started taking doula trainings and workshops around perinatal mental health, and I started learning about trauma-informed care and harm reduction and pulling bits and pieces from all of these different learning tools to share with my doula clients. My clients were primarily unhoused folks who also were struggling with community and with their sense of self, and I was just having conversations with them about that: What does it mean to have community?

C3 Care is a process for folks to explore where they are at, what they need, what is around them for support and resources, and how they can engage with the people and places in their community. It is intended for folks who are solo parenting, partnered in parenting, new parents, seasoned parents, and intended parents.

It is a three-step process that focuses on self-reflection (what do I need?), environmental survey (what resources are available?), and accountability and consent (how can I make a plan with my community?). The care model is based on three "C" words:

1. **Conscious.** The first step involves defining your wellness through internal reflection to know what support you need from others.

2. **Compassion.** The second step is to build a community map and do an environmental survey. This step is about nurturing authentic community connections and learning about the resources, supports, and people available to you. We need to do this work so that when we feel alone, we know where we can go for help.

3. **Collective.** The third step revolves around accountability and boundaries. This is about building collective understanding of expectations, identifying your boundaries and those of other people in your community. How will you navigate holding others accountable when they say they will help, how will you make sure you have the same ideas of what help looks like? This step is about setting expectations for yourself and others.

C3 care is not a quick fix. It took me years to say I actually have a community. This is why when I talk about community building, it's always in terms of "the sooner the better." Don't wait until you are pregnant or after your kiddo arrives — this is a long game. Community building is an active and engaging practice, and it took me that long because I'd started with nothing. The C3 Care model recognizes the need for ongoing care and support, not just during the immediate postpartum period but throughout the parenting journey.

A lot of the people I was friends with prior to becoming a parent, I do not talk to anymore, and a lot of the people who are now closest to me have entered my life more recently. I was able to build these foundational relationships and connections because I finally understood who I was and what I actually needed, and I actually knew what my boundaries were.

LHZ: We wait to start building a community or we think it is a problem for "future us." We don't start thinking about what we need until we need it. But you are talking about starting an ongoing process because when you need your community it's not the right time to build your community. We need to start now.

GG: Start now and open up conversations about the future and your needs. I've seen beautiful, beautiful ways that folks have communicated their needs and also prepared for the challenges that they might encounter. You know, sometimes it's just a straight up phone call to talk about support: "This is what's going on. I'm going to be going through this pregnancy and I'm at risk for PMADS [perinatal or postpartum mood and anxiety disorder]. These are the signs of depression for me. Currently, I'm imagining the symptoms are going to be very similar, but they might be different. These are things my healthcare provider shared. If you notice these symptoms, this is what would be helpful." It's about having those really raw, very vulnerable conversations and asking clearly for help.

We think that family, chosen family, friends are going to know how to be there in the ways that are meaningful for us, but if you don't actually talk about it, they may not know what to look for or what support you need. We need to do this work intentionally before the postpartum period because it takes time and conversation. The more we prepare, the more clarity we have for ourselves around what sustains our wellness, what we need from external sources to sustain that wellness, and the conversations we need to have to make a direct and clear ask from our community.

LHZ: So often, there's a disconnect around what support looks like for each of us, if we don't have those intentional conversations. It sounds like your goal in working with people is to help them think about what care looks like, what accountability looks like, and what consent-based community looks like.

GG: Unfortunately, sometimes the people that we want specific care from (including partners) aren't able to show up in the ways we'd hoped, which is why it is so important to have these conversations before getting pregnant or building a family. Whenever possible, having these discussions in advance is essential, because there may be some shock and grieving around how you expect a person to show up and how they envision it or what they are prepared for. When we engage in this as a preventative care approach or sustainable care approach, we need to allot time to process that and potentially find other people and places to fill in those gaps, because you still have the needs that need to be met.

LHZ: I can see how these conversations would be applicable to trying to conceive as well. Even thinking about supporting someone going through an IVF process or an experience of loss. If you don't have conversations in advance about how you want or need to be cared for, then you're not going to be able to show up for each other in meaningful ways. We don't want to talk about worst-case scenarios because they are scary. We worry that somehow talking about them might make them more real or more possible. But if we have conversations about what would feel supportive in times of grief or physical hardship, then we can be there for each other or find other people who can be there for us.

GG: Exactly. Thinking about partners and family: your partner, as a whole person, is also going through this new parenting experience or grieving experience, and they may also have childhood trauma triggers. You may feel like, "You're my person, so you're supposed to help me as my person and do these things or that." But they just may not be able to give what you need for whatever reason or be able to show up in the way that you expected them to, and you didn't communicate what that looks like for each of you.

LHZ: Why are these conversations so important for 2SLGBTQ+ families?

GG: Queer and trans families sometimes look different from more normative families. So, if you've been navigating life with a chosen family and there are no babies around them yet — you might have friends' dinners every week, or you might be hanging out all the time in a bar or social setting — and then suddenly, things shift with a baby and there can sometimes be a disconnect with your community. And that can feel lonely. Our families look different from normative families, so there are more conversations about what we imagine our futures to be. I think there are a lot of reasons for why that happens, but it shows that there is a real need for conversation and expectation setting.

It might involve conversations like, "Hey, I have a clinic appointment today, I'm feeling really nervous about it, can you come with me?" or "I'm having big emotions about this procedure" or "I'm really excited about this thing, can I call you after?" It might be decompressing with a close person after being misgendered at a clinic or having to pay for mandated counselling with a therapist you don't know. It is so important to have people in your corner who can attend to your specific needs.

The C3 model of care is built around activities and guided self-reflections in the beginning. The first C is really a lot of journaling conversations with self and conversations with partners and chosen family. There is also a lot of vulnerability with this work as well. You could spend twenty minutes doing self-reflection, or you could spend forever. You could take weeks or months to really reflect and process where you're at right now before even trying to do an environmental scan of resources available.

The second part is really focusing on what resources and spaces are available to you now, during pregnancy, postpartum, and in parenting. Do you see yourself bringing your baby into community spaces? Are they accessible? Do they have other people like you and your family? If your current social life is very active in the evening and you like to go out and socialize and have drinks and go to the bars, that's great. Is that a space that you want to bring your baby? If you do, cool. If you don't, what are the things that you can do now to start to shift your environment and engage with other communities in spaces where you do want to bring your baby. Because if you wait until you have the baby you could be stuck in the house. You could experience a shift in hormones and emotions, and you could feel very alone and disconnected: "What do I do? Where do I go?"

For queer community as well, suss it out, check out the vibes. Is that community centre welcoming? Is that play group actually a place you want to bring your baby? Ask questions of the community; check out different online groups to find people like you and your family. Doing this environmental scan is about identifying the support that will help in the areas that you need. The third C is when you seek consent and communicate your needs. If you already struggle to get chores done or to get through laundry, make a plan for when you are doing IVF or when you are expecting, or after the baby arrives. Reach out to friends and family: "Are these things that you would be down to help me with when the baby's here?" There's so many different ways that people can help you with particular tasks that feel overwhelming; some friends might do your laundry, others might help with a laundry service or hiring a cleaning person, or bringing you meals. Planning ahead gives people the opportunity to show up in the ways that they want to and that will allow it to feel sustainable, caring, and reciprocal for both of you.

C3 Care is about being clear about what you need. It's a domino effect of doing the internal reflection, then external reflection, and then communicating with the people around you about what you've been processing and reflecting on.

LHZ: It's amazing how, when preparing for postpartum, so much resonates with preparing to try to make a baby. There are so many times when your mental health is at risk, or you feel alone, or you need support. So, preparing for these things in advance, you learn about mental health for the future and for right now. These are tools that help you to build community in meaningful ways — not just friendships, but really meaningful communities for every stage of the process. Do you think there are specific barriers for 2SLGBTQ+ people in this process?

GG: I see that people in the queer and transgender community are always held to this different standard, or asked questions that other families aren't asked: "Are you sure that you want this baby?" And it's like, "Yes, I am sure!" There are extra barriers or hoops that we have to jump through.

One of the barriers I see is that in healthcare training, 2SLGBTQ+ people are only talked about for thirty minutes, and it's not integrated into the curriculum. It's this special course on the side or extra professional development. People accessing care have to teach their providers and it's tiresome and feels like erasure. Trans folks exploring family building — whether they're the birthing partner or not — have to repeatedly explain their identities. I've had clients in the past share that their doctors didn't understand why they needed sperm — because this person passed as male — and the doctors weren't reading their chart. The barriers are extensive. The spaces that folks go to do IVF or IUI are very, very, very, very, very gendered and there is always an assumption that something is "wrong."

I hope that leaders and peers in the field continue to speak up and advocate, and we get more information out there that shows that it really isn't that different. Parenting is parenting and showing up for a child is showing up for a child. We end up feeling so othered and there is just all this bullshit — I'm sorry I don't have another word for it — that folks experience that breaks my heart every single time. It is deeply homophobic for anyone to demand that you convince them of your right to have a baby. That is why I feel so grateful to be witnessing everything happening through Seed and Sprout at Birth Mark. Seeing the ways that community members show up for one another, it's one of the most heartwarming things. Queer community is so incredibly skilled at navigating barriers and supporting others to get through those barriers, and I do hope that with more information, there's more space for us to just take up, where we don't have to advocate and overexplain. It would be beautiful for people to just exist.

STEPS TO BUILD YOUR

COMMUNITY MAP

01 — WHO DO YOU KNOW ?

MAKE A LIST OF EVERYONE YOU KNOW. FRIENDS, FAMILY, CO-WORKERS, ACQUAINTENCES. THE BIGGER THE LIST THE BETTER.

02 — HOW CAN THEY SUPPORT?

NOW THAT YOU KNOW WHAT YOUR NEEDS ARE, ASK YOURSELF: HOW CAN THE PEOPLE ON THIS LIST HELP YOU ACCOMPLISH THIS?

03 — REACH OUT, ASK FOR HELP

YEAH, THIS PART. YOU HAVE TO STEP UP AND ASK FOR WHAT YOU NEED. THIS PART MAY NEED SOME PRACTICE.

4.
Understanding Our Parts

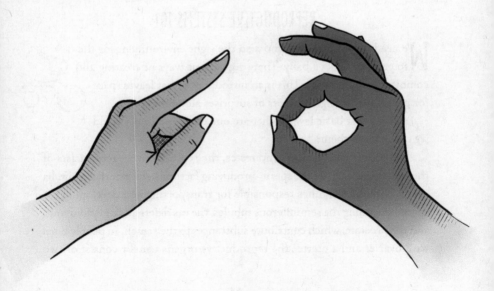

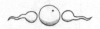

This part is about reproductive systems, cycles, gamete (sperm and egg) development, common conditions, and hormones. The next pages share more information about the body parts and hormones that help make conception possible, the things that you might not remember from a sex-ed class (or maybe never learned about at all), as well as common conditions and diagnostic tools that help to identify when there might be barriers or other considerations in planning your family-building journey. Read this part if you are curious to learn more about your body or the bodies that might help you to conceive.

REPRODUCTIVE SYSTEMS 101

We need sperm and eggs and also the right environment for them to grow to make a baby. There are various ways of creating and combining these things. This is an introduction that leaves space for possibility, change, and lots of surprises along the way.

At the most basic level: What are our parts and how should we check in on them?

For people with penises and testes, the reproductive tract consists of the testicles, which are the sperm-producing factories, the external genitalia (penis), and all the tubes responsible for transporting and developing the sperm, including the seminiferous tubules, the vas deferens, the epididymis, and the prostate, which contribute substances to the semen. In people born with ovaries and a uterus, the reproductive organs usually consist of two ovaries, which produce eggs, and the fallopian tubes, which connect the ovaries to the uterus. The uterus is responsible for the growth of the endometrium (or uterine lining) and its shedding during a menstrual cycle, causing bleeding.

For people with any of these parts, these systems are controlled by the brain — specifically the hypothalamus and pituitary, which secrete hormones that signal to the testes or the ovaries to produce sperm or eggs.

Taking care of your body is about being in tune with your needs, being kind to yourself, and responding to cues your body might be telling you if something is a little off. For people with ovaries and eggs, that might look like tracking symptoms or the timing of your menstrual cycle with an app or calendar. Pay attention: Are they consistent? Long? Short? Very heavy? Very light? Painful? Let your body give you insight into how it is doing. Your body is telling you a story every month, and it's always developing and changing. Keep track of your cycles and talk to a doctor if things feel a little (or a lot!) off. Basic fertility testing with a fertility clinic or testing and conversations with a naturopath or acupuncturist can start to give you deeper insight into your reproductive health.

For people with sperm, listening to your body is equally important (but sometimes a bit harder to track). Watch for any changes to your body, like loss of energy, change in libido, or erectile dysfunction. See a reproductive specialist if you are struggling to conceive or are concerned about your reproductive health. Provincial healthcare often covers semen analysis for those trying to conceive or thinking about conception in their future. There are now also apps and at-home tests that you can do (at a cost), using a smartphone camera or an at-home kit, to test basic parameters for sperm. While these cover only certain factors, it is a window into your body that might be a good starting place if you are curious about your sperm.

ABOUT EGGS

Gametes are the specialized cells (sperm and eggs) that are involved in human reproduction, and can combine during fertilization to form a zygote, which can develop into an embryo and then can grow into fetus, and then a baby.

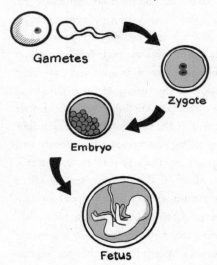

Gametes

Zygote

Embryo

Fetus

For people with ovaries, the reproductive system produces eggs (also called oocytes) through a process of oogenesis. It begins during fetal development in utero. Amazingly, babies are born with all the eggs they will ever have, already present in the ovaries at the time of birth. That means that the egg that would become you was inside of your parent, when they were inside of your grandparent. Bodies are incredible.

The oocytes that a fetus is born with are arrested at birth and stop growing until the onset of puberty, when hormonal changes in the body trigger the release of primary oocytes. Then during each menstrual cycle, typically one primary oocyte resumes development and matures each month (more on that next).

If someone is on gender-affirming hormone therapy (GAHT), the impact on ovulatory function is reversible when GAHT is discontinued and it does not impact clinical pregnancy rates. After stopping therapy, ovulatory function usually resumes and the menstrual cycle typically returns after a few months. If there are underlying conditions, irregular periods, polycystic ovary syndrome (PCOS), endometriosis, or low ovarian reserve, just like anyone else with eggs, this may impact your fertility.

MENSTRUAL CYCLES

Understanding menstrual cycles helps us to understand reproduction, some conditions or diagnoses we might receive in the journey, and how and why some protocols might be recommended. We often aren't taught about our bodies or forget the lessons we learn because they are taught in ways that feel distant, irrelevant, or uncomfortable.

The Menstrual Cycle

The menstrual cycle is a cyclic process (typically occurring monthly) based on hormonal shifts in the body. Each month if someone with ovaries and a uterus has a regular period and no underlying conditions, their body will grow an egg (follicular phase), ovulate (ovulatory phase), and continue to go through a series of hormonal shifts to support potential pregnancy (luteal phase), until a fertilized egg implants or (if one doesn't) the next period begins. Typically, this cycle takes between twenty-five and thirty-five days (counting from the beginning of the bleeding [cycle day 1] to the first day of the next bleed).

Not all bodies with a uterus and ovaries do these steps at the same intervals and not all bodies do them at all. If you do not menstruate, if you do not menstruate frequently, or if there are other irregularities, this does not mean you cannot get pregnant or carry a baby. It *may* mean you need a little support or intervention, or it may mean that it could take a little longer.

During your period, there are changes happening in your ovaries and in your uterus. Let's break down what is going on each step of the way.

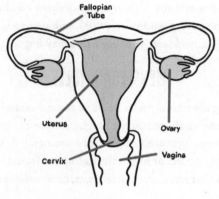

Fallopian
Tube

Uterus

Ovary

Cervix

Vagina

In the Ovaries

Days 1–14: On the first day of your period, the hormones from your brain cause a number of your eggs (inside of sacs called follicles) to start growing in your ovaries, until one follicle takes the lead and becomes "dominant."

Day 14: Around day 14 (though it is different for all bodies and can shift each month based on a number of factors) that one dominant follicle releases a mature egg. This process is triggered by a surge in luteinizing hormone (LH). The released egg enters the fallopian tube. If you are trying to conceive, this is where fertilization typically occurs if sperm is present. The egg is viable for fertilization for about twelve to twenty-four hours.

Days 15–28: This is called the luteal phase. After ovulation, the ruptured follicle (that sac that the egg popped out of) transforms into a structure called the corpus luteum. The corpus luteum produces hormones, primarily progesterone, to prepare the uterus for a pregnancy.

In the Uterus

Days 1–5: When you start your period, your uterine lining sheds from the last cycle.

Days 6–14: Because of increasing hormones (mostly estrogen) at this stage, the uterus starts building a new lining in preparation for a potential pregnancy.

Days 15–28: Called the secretory phase, the uterus continues to grow thicker lining to support a potential pregnancy. This lining will shed on your day 1 of the next cycle if you are not pregnant.

And Now a Little More Detail....

If you want to understand the hormones at play during a menstrual cycle (and maybe get a sense of what some IVF medications are trying to do) read this next section. It is a little bit of a biology lesson and hopefully will give you new ways to think about your body!

There are a few major functional components that support and shape your reproduction and menstrual cycle. The HPO axis (composed of the hypothalamus, pituitary, and ovaries) and the thyroid and uterus play important roles in our cycles and how they progress. Situated centrally in the brain, the hypothalamus engages in communication with the pituitary gland through a blood exchange. Within the hypothalamus, which is a kind of control centre, various hormones are generated. One crucial hormone essential for reproduction is gonadotropin-releasing hormone (GnRH), released by the hypothalamus, that sets off a cascade of hormonal events crucial for ovulation, fertilization, and the preparation of the uterine lining.

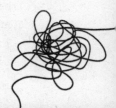

Menstruation

When you start your period, your estrogen levels (produced primarily by your ovaries) are low. You shed your lining from the previous cycle. In your brain, the hypothalamus is stimulated to produce GnRH, which stimulates the anterior pituitary gland to produce luteinizing hormone (LH) and follicle-stimulating hormone (FSH), which are both important to follicular growth and ovulation. These two hormones are called gonadotropins. They are essential for getting your eggs to grow before you ovulate. As these follicles develop, they release estrogen, which will 1) help your endometrium (lining of uterus) to get thicker to prepare for potential implantation of an embryo, and 2) cause your cervical mucus to get thinner, clear, and watery to potentially facilitate sperm to move more easily.

Development from an initial tiny follicle (called a primordial follicle) to dominant follicle (the one that you will ovulate at the end of the month), actually takes about three to four menstrual cycles. So, the egg that you ovulate has been growing for months before ovulation. This is why it is often suggested to start taking prenatal vitamins a few months before you are ready to conceive (don't worry if you haven't started yet! But it doesn't hurt to get a head start).

Once a dominant follicle matures it produces high levels of estrogen that send a message to the pituitary to produce a surge (sudden increase) of LH and that triggers ovulation — the LH surge facilitates the final maturation and release of the oocyte (egg) from the follicle.

The LH surge is key to discerning your timing for conception. You can often determine when it occurs from a urine test or bloodwork. After ovulation, when the follicle releases an egg, the ruptured follicle transforms into a structure called the corpus luteum, which produces progesterone.

That progesterone, along with estrogen, helps maintain the thick lining of the uterus, which you need in order for a potential embryo to implant in the wall of the uterus. You need both the embryo and the optimal environment for it to be ready for embryo development and support. That corpus luteum will produce estrogen for fourteen days, after which (if the person does not conceive) it will stop. The declining estrogen and progesterone will tell your body that the lining will no longer be needed, and you will begin to shed the lining of your uterus (a menstruation!) and the next cycle begins.

IVF Transfers and the Corpus Luteum

When we talk about options for IVF transfers, I explain what a "programmed" cycle is. Since you don't ovulate in these cycles, there is no corpus luteum. While you will take progesterone after any IVF transfer, this medication plays an especially important role after a programmed cycle, because it takes on the job of the absent corpus luteum.

CHARTING YOUR CYCLE

If you have a uterus and eggs and you are planning to try to conceive at home, one thing you likely need to do is determine when you will ovulate. Right before you ovulate is when you are most fertile, and the two to three days prior to ovulation are when you want to try to conceive.

In full transparency, I find tracking cycles a bit tricky, and the charts and instructions can sometimes feel overwhelming. For me (and maybe for some of you reading this), it is beneficial to know that there is more than one way to track your cycle, a bit of it is trial and error, and often it is by using a combination of methods that feel right for you that will give you the best indication of when you ovulate.

Menstrual Cycle

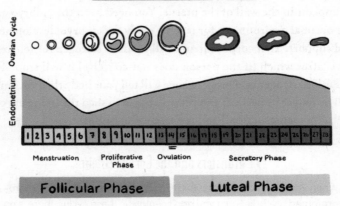

Ovarian Cycle

Endometrium

| 1 2 3 4 5 6 7 8 9 10 11 12 13 14 15 16 17 18 19 20 21 22 23 24 25 26 27 28 |

Menstruation   Proliferative   Ovulation   Secretory Phase
                Phase

Follicular Phase   **Luteal Phase**

If you do not ovulate at regular intervals, you may need the help of a fertility clinic to either help you track when you ovulate or, if you don't do so on your own, prescribe medications to help your body to ovulate. Acupuncturists and naturopaths are also options that can potentially support ovulation.

Because some of the best signs you have ovulated only occur *after* you ovulate, a lot of this is prep work before you try to conceive. You need to be tracking for at least three months to really get a sense of your cycle and to understand how predictable it is. So, start planning and tracking well in advance from when you want to try to conceive.

Overview of Options for Cycle Charting

1. **Cycle monitoring at a fertility clinic.** A clinic can do bloodwork and ultrasounds to get the most exact timing of ovulation based on your hormones and follicular development.

2. **LH strips or ovulation predictor kits.** These are tests you pee on that look for an LH surge, which would indicate that ovulation is happening. These are not very useful for people with PCOS, for whom LH levels do not always follow a predictable or expected pattern.

3. **Basal body temperature (BBT).** This is your temperature when your body is fully at rest. It has to be taken, using a BBT thermometer or a wearable BBT tracking device, in the morning before you get out of bed or move around. Tracking the slight rise in body temperature can help you determine when you ovulate.

4. **Cervical position.** Using a finger to feel for your cervix can help you determine when you ovulate since your cervix will shift and open or close based on where you are in your cycle.

5. **Cervical mucus (or discharge).** Your cervical mucus tells you a lot about where you are in your cycle and can be a great tool to get a sense of when you ovulate.

How to Check Your Cervix

Checking the cervical position takes some practice. To check your cervix, wash your hands and trim nails. Often people find sitting on the toilet, standing with one leg elevated on a bathtub, or squatting to be good positions. To be able to feel the shifts in your cervix over your cycle, use the same position each time you check. Insert one or two fingers into the vaginal opening and feel the upper front or top to find the cervix. Depending on where you are in your cycle, it might feel like the tip of a nose or as soft as a lip or earlobe. Its firmness and openness will change based on where you are in your cycle.

Next is a breakdown of how your BBT, cervix position, and cervical mucus all shift throughout your cycle. You can also use an app to track the information you gather, but I would caution against assuming a calendar app knows when you are ovulating based only on tracking your menstrual cycle. These apps will generally assume your body ovulates on day 14 of your cycle and that is not always the case.

Pre-ovulation Phase (Follicular Phase)

BBT. During the first half of your cycle (around days 1–14), before ovulation occurs, your temperature tends to remain relatively low, typically ranging from around 97°F to 97.5°F. You're looking for a baseline temperature pattern during this phase, noting any fluctuations that could indicate hormonal changes leading up to ovulation.

Cervical mucus. In the first 1 to 4 day(s) after menstrual bleeding, cervical mucus is typically thick and dry or tacky. The colour may be white or tinged yellow. Over the course of your follicular phase, as estrogen rises, cervical mucus production increases. The mucus becomes more abundant, going from sticky and opaque on days 4–6 to wet and cloudy (like yogurt) on days 7–9. By days 10–14 it will become slippery, wet, and clear, similar to raw egg whites.

Cervical position. During menstrual bleeding, the cervix is typically hard, low, and slightly open in order to allow blood to be released. Following menstruation, the cervix gradually rises higher in the vaginal canal and can feel firm, slightly open, or closed. Often people say it feels like the tip of your nose. When estrogen levels rise, leading up to ovulation, the cervix gets softer, more open, and higher up.

Ovulation Phase

BBT. For some people, just before ovulation, there is a slight *drop* in BBT, followed by a rise in temperature after ovulation occurs. That sharp increase indicates ovulation. The temperature rise is caused by the increase in progesterone, and it usually ranges from about 0.4°F to 1.0°F and can last the remainder of your cycle, until your next period. You're looking for this sustained temperature increase, so if your temperature has risen and remains steady for three or more days, this serves as a strong indicator that ovulation has already taken place.

The reason we need to chart in advance is because your most fertile days are approximately two days before your basal body temperature rises — your goal is to try to conceive just before you ovulate, and the rise in temperature indicates that ovulation has already occurred.

Cervical mucus. As you approach ovulation and reach peak fertility, your cervical mucus will look like raw egg whites (clear, slippery, transparent). You will have the most mucus at this time. Bodies are prepping for potential conception, as this fertile cervical mucus will help sperm move through the cervix into the uterus.

Cervical position. Around ovulation, the cervix is usually at its highest position and feels soft, moist, and open — like touching an earlobe or a lip. For some people it can be so high, it can be hard to reach.

Post-ovulation Phase (Luteal Phase)

BBT. After ovulation, your BBT remains elevated compared to the pre-ovulation phase. If pregnancy does not occur, your BBT will generally stay elevated for about ten to fourteen days before dropping again, just before the start of your next menstrual period.

Cervical mucus. Post-ovulation, as estrogen levels decrease, there is also a decrease in cervical mucus. Some people experience dryness in this period, others just have a small amount of thicker or sticker mucus.

Cervical position. Following ovulation, the cervix moves lower in the vaginal canal and again becomes firmer and more closed — this can happen right when you ovulate or can take a few hours or even days for some people. As progesterone levels rise, cervical mucus production decreases and the cervix may feel drier.

ABOUT SPERM

Sperm refers to reproductive cells (gametes) in most people born with testes and a penis. They are produced in the testes through a process called *spermatogenesis*. Not all people produce sperm and not all sperm works in the same way. When tests analyze sperm, the most basic aspects evaluate *sperm count*, or the concentration of sperm in a given amount of semen; *sperm motility*, or how they move; and *sperm morphology*, or the shape and structure of the sperm. At some clinics, doctors will also suggest DNA fragmentation tests, particularly for people with infertility/recurrent pregnancy loss, failure with IVF or intracytoplasmic sperm injection (ICSI), or other clinical symptoms. DNA fragmentation tests often mean an additional fee and is not recommended as a routine test for all patients. There are other tests that can be done on sperm as well, but these are the basics.

If you produce sperm and are considering GAHT, it is preferable to freeze sperm before starting feminizing hormone treatment when possible. If for some reason you cannot or did not preserve sperm before starting GAHT, that doesn't necessarily mean that you cannot produce sperm if you stop in the future. There is a common assumption (among medical professionals) that the impact of GAHT on spermatogenesis inhibition is irreversible. There weren't strong studies to support this in the past. However, a 2023 longitudinal study (de Nie et al.) on transgender women undergoing GAHT found that spermatogenesis inhibition might not be permanent. It was a small study looking at nine transgender women and more work needs to be done, but they found that all nine women who discontinued GAHT for reproductive reasons had viable sperm. The women in the study were between eighteen and thirty-two years old and were using GAHT for a range of 6 to 216 months (median was thirty-six months). Following cessation of GAHT, viable sperm were eventually documented in all nine cases. Of those in the study, four participants stopped GAHT to conceive, and five stopped to bank sperm for potential future use. So, while this study was not a sizable sample, it does tell us something really important: contrary to common belief, hormone treatment for trans women does not necessarily result in permanent infertility. We need more studies to get more information.

SPERM DEVELOPMENT AND MATURATION
Initiation of Sperm Development

Sperm development starts at puberty in the testes when the hypothalamus releases GnRH, stimulating the pituitary gland to release FSH and LH into the bloodstream. Yes! These are the same kinds of hormones that are supporting the development of eggs and impacting the menstrual cycle. From the bloodstream, FSH and LH travel to the testes. Here, FSH plays a key role in stimulating the production of immature sperm cells, called spermatogonia. LH plays a crucial role here, too, by stimulating the Leydig cells in the testes to produce testosterone.

Testosterone is a key hormone for maturation of immature sperm cells into fully developed and functional sperm cells. So, in basic terms: FSH stimulates the production of immature sperm cells, while LH stimulates the production of testosterone, which supports spermatogenesis.

Inside the testes, the immature spermatogonia continue to develop into spermatozoa (mature sperm) and travel to a coiled tube in the penis called the epididymis. We can think about the movement through the epididymis like going to a university campus for sperm — it is where they go to learn to swim and gain the ability to fertilize eggs. In the epididymis, the sperm go through further maturation and are stored there until they are ready to be ejaculated.

The process of sperm maturation, from the initial development of sperm cells to their full maturation, typically takes about seventy-four days (two and a half to three months). This duration is based on the various stages of spermatogenesis. So, the sperm you use today will have been growing for a few months before making their way to an egg!

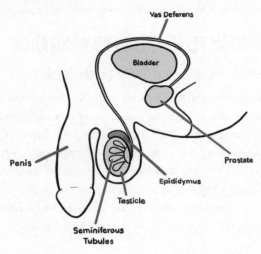

DIAGNOSTIC TESTING

If you are planning to build your family, there are a number of diagnostic tests you (and/or your donor, partner, or surrogate) might choose to undergo. Some of these tests (like bloodwork for hormone levels, thyroid levels, or STIs) can be done by a family doctor, walk-in clinic, or sexual health clinic. Other tests may require you to go to a fertility specialist or a fertility clinic (like an internal ultrasound or sonohysterogram). If you are working with a fertility clinic, they will likely have procedural diagnostic tests they will ask you or your partner to undergo. If you are concerned, have questions, or are unsure if a test is medically necessary, you can always ask the care provider which tests are optional, which are required by their clinic due to internal policies, and which are required by Health Canada. Any testing required by Health Canada is likely non-negotiable.

Broadly, if you, a donor, or a co-parent produce sperm, they will initially do a sperm analysis and blood test. If you, a donor, or a co-parent have eggs and a uterus, they will likely do bloodwork and an internal ultrasound. They may also look at your uterus and fallopian tubes. Below is a more comprehensive list of some of the initial tests that provide insight into your body, hormones, and fertility.

For People with Eggs and Uterus (Including Donors and Some for Surrogates)

+ STI testing
+ Follicle-stimulating hormone (FSH) (blood test)
+ Anti-Müllerian hormone (AMH) (blood test)
+ Antral follicle count (AFC) (internal ultrasound)

+ Uterine and/or fallopian tube testing: an X-ray to check if fallopian tubes are open and the uterine cavity is normal

+ Thyroid function testing (blood test)

+ Genetic screening; depending on family history, carrier screening for genetic disorders (blood test)

+ Some clinics will ask that you be up to date on pap smears prior to beginning treatments

For People with Sperm (Including Donors)

+ Semen analysis to assess sperm count, motility, morphology, and other characteristics

+ Hormone testing: testosterone, follicle-stimulating hormone (FSH), luteinizing hormone (LH) (blood test)

+ Infectious disease screening: tests for STIs and infections that might impact sperm health (blood test)

+ Genetic screening; depending on family history, carrier screening for genetic disorders (blood test)

+ Physical examination to check for abnormalities or conditions affecting reproductive organs

Hormonal Evaluation

A blood test is done to measure hormone levels (follicle-stimulating hormone [FSH], luteinizing hormone [LH], estrogen, progesterone, and thyroid hormones). These tests will give your doctor insight into ovarian function and hormonal balance and help them to design a protocol and plan that best fits your body.

Ovarian Reserve Testing

A blood test will also assess your "ovarian reserve" or anti-Müllerian hormone (AMH) levels. AMH is a protein hormone produced by the cells in the ovaries. Because it provides information on the quantity of remaining eggs, sometimes this test is called a "fertility test." Some companies might sell it privately and say that they are assessing your fertility. The problem is that available evidence indicates that AMH levels do not effectively predict a person's current or future fertility very well. The test gives some insight into the number of eggs remaining, but it does not offer a comprehensive understanding of someone's fertility, information on the quality of their eggs, or the rate at which their egg count will decrease. It is one piece of a much larger puzzle. We currently don't have a way to test egg *quality*, though we know that egg quality typically will decline with age. If your AMH levels come back low, remember: this does not tell us anything about your ability to conceive right now. These numbers are just one part of the picture and don't define your fertility. Talk to your doctor about their recommendations and don't be afraid to get a second opinion if you require more information.

Thyroid Testing

The thyroid is a butterfly-shaped gland in your neck that regulates metabolism and (among other things) controls how quickly the body uses energy and makes protein. The gland is in continuous communication with the ovaries, and thyroid hormones play a significant role in various stages of reproduction. In the context of fertility, thyroid dysfunctions are relatively common and can have diverse impacts on reproduction such as anovulatory cycles (not ovulating), elevated prolactin levels, and imbalances in sex hormones. When thyroid disorders go undiagnosed and untreated, they can become a potential cause of infertility or losses, affecting a person's ability to conceive or maintain a pregnancy. People who have irregular menstrual cycles may have bloodwork done to check thyroid function, as irregularities in the thyroid can impact your cycle.

Ultrasound Tests

An internal ultrasound will give your doctor a clearer image of your internal reproductive organs. The following ultrasound tests may be used throughout fertility treatment and can help answer many questions.

Antral follicle count. During your internal ultrasound, the technician will be counting the number of follicles that they see in your ovaries. A lower follicle count may suggest diminished ovarian reserve, while a count high above the typical range for your age may be one potential indication of polycystic ovarian syndrome. It is normal for younger people to have a higher AFC than people who are older. Your ovarian reserve does go down as you age.

Sonohysterogram (uterine cavity assessment). Some clinics will routinely suggest a sonohysterogram, a diagnostic examination that helps your physician assess the inside of the uterus. During this procedure, a small amount of saline solution is inserted into the uterine cavity, helping the doctor to visualize the uterus through a transvaginal ultrasound. Sonohysterograms are typically performed following the conclusion of menstruation but before ovulation, which typically falls within days 5 to 11 of the menstrual cycle. Some people experience light cramping during the procedure, others experience high levels of pain. Ask your doctor or nurse about pain medications to help manage any discomfort, pain, or anxiety.

Diagnostic Cycle

Your clinic might do a kind of "practice" or "diagnostic" cycle for people using their eggs/uterus. Not every clinic suggests this step and you can ask them to skip it (or why they recommend it) if that is your preference. In this process, they watch your cycle to see how you progress and what your body does naturally or without medication. They do a full cycle (a month) without insemination, retrieval of eggs, or transfer of embryos, just to see what your body does.

If your clinic doesn't do a diagnostic cycle, the stage after testing is to secure whatever gametes you need (sperm or eggs) and to move forward with cycle monitoring followed by either IUI or egg retrieval.

COMMON CONDITIONS
For People with Sperm

For individuals with sperm, there are a number of conditions and external factors that can influence sperm quality, motility, and mobility. Lifestyle choices, like smoking and recreational drug use (especially anabolic steroids), can impact sperm parameters — sometimes these have long-term impacts and sometimes they can be corrected or improved over time. Excessive alcohol consumption, STIs, and enlarged veins in the testicles (varicocele) are other factors that can affect sperm production and quality. Genetic abnormalities, advanced age, stress, heat exposure to the testicles, nutrient deficiencies, and stress also play a role in sperm health. Medical treatments like chemotherapy and radiation, as well as certain medications, can harm sperm production. Ask your fertility specialist, doctor, or naturopath if you have questions about your body or think that these factors might be influencing your attempts to conceive.

For People with Uteruses, Ovaries, and Eggs

Amenorrhea. This is the clinical name for not getting your period and there are two main types:

- **Primary:** when someone hasn't had their first period by age sixteen or within five years of puberty.

- **Secondary:** when someone has been having regular periods but stops getting them for more than three months. Hypothalamic amenorrhea, also called functional hypothalamic amenorrhea or FHA, is a condition where someone doesn't have their period due to an issue with the hypothalamus in the brain. The hypothalamus controls things like body temperature, hunger, and parts of reproduction by releasing GnRH. When the hypothalamus stops making enough GnRH, it interferes with the balance of hormones, leading to irregular or absent periods. FHA affects around 17.4 million people globally (Shufelt and Dutra 2017).

PCOS. Polycystic ovary syndrome (PCOS) is a common disorder that affects people with ovaries. One of the most common symptoms of PCOS is an elevated number of follicles in the ovaries. In individuals *without* PCOS, the ovarian cycle typically follows a pattern where one follicle becomes dominant and matures each month, eventually leading to monthly ovulation of a single egg. However, in people with PCOS, abnormal hormone levels prevent normal maturation or release of the egg. Instead, the immature follicles accumulate in the ovaries, which can prevent regular ovulation.

While the exact cause of PCOS is not fully understood, it is believed to involve a combination of genetic and environmental factors that impact hormone levels, particularly an excess of androgens (like testosterone) leading to irregular menstrual cycles. Common symptoms of PCOS include irregular periods, ovarian cysts, acne, excessive hair growth, and sometimes weight gain. Not every individual with PCOS will experience all these symptoms and their severity may vary. If you get testing from a fertility clinic, high levels of AMH and "polycystic ovaries" (meaning many follicles are seen on an internal ultrasound) are other signs of PCOS. People with PCOS may require medical intervention in order to conceive, though not all do. Naturopathic doctors may be able to help in managing PCOS, if a person prefers to try to regulate hormones outside of a fertility clinic, or with additional support.

In Canada, there are an estimated 1.4 million people who may have PCOS (though this number may be impacted by a lack of diagnostic tests performed or by underreporting). The World Health Organization (2023a) estimates that PCOS affects an estimated 8–13 percent of reproductive-aged people with ovaries and that up to 70 percent of those affected remain undiagnosed worldwide. In their 2023 study, Ismayilova and Yaya note that "many women feel that they do not receive sufficient information about their condition and are frustrated by the limited knowledge of PCOS they find in professionals and their inconsistent approaches to diagnosis and management of PCOS. Studies of healthcare providers found that many may need more knowledge on PCOS and have a limited amount of information available for patients about PCOS and its management" (2023: 57). So, while PCOS is one of the most common conditions that can impact monthly cycles, pain, and fertility, it is poorly understood, undertreated, and underdiagnosed. Like many conditions impacting people with ovaries, individuals with PCOS report needing to educate themselves, gather their own resources, and advocate for their needs (Ismayilova and Yaya 2023).

PCOS can impact fertility in a number of ways, including the following:

+ Irregular ovulation or the lack of ovulation (anovulation). A fertility clinic or doctor can prescribe medications to support ovulation.

+ Elevated levels of androgens in PCOS can disrupt the normal hormonal balance necessary for a regular menstrual cycle. People with PCOS often have irregular or very long menstrual cycles with heavy bleeding. These hormonal imbalances can affect the maturation and release of eggs from the ovaries.

+ Some individuals with PCOS have insulin resistance, which may contribute to hormonal imbalances and interfere with normal ovarian function.

+ Individuals report feeling unheard and being undertreated by healthcare professionals, which can impact mental health.

Endometriosis. This is a condition where tissue similar to the lining of the uterus grows outside the uterus and has no way to leave the body. Endometriosis has different levels of severity and can affect ovaries, fallopian tubes, and the tissue lining the pelvis. This can cause pain, scar tissue, and adhesions. Not everyone with endometriosis will experience infertility. But for some, treatments can help them to conceive (and relieve some of the painful symptoms). The most apparent symptom for endometriosis is painful periods. Some people experience pain during vaginal penetration, during bowel movements, or irregular bleeding between cycles. But some people experience no symptoms at all! Endometriosis is hard to diagnose because doing so is generally only possible with invasive laparoscopic surgery (which some clinics and doctors are hesitant to provide). Because of this, it is likely more common than we think and may often go undiagnosed, or symptoms are ignored by individuals or their providers.

GENDER-AFFIRMING HORMONES AND FAMILY-FORMING CONSIDERATIONS

by A.J. Lowik

A.J. Lowik is an assistant professor at the University of Lethbridge and a re-searcher and activist in transgender reproductive rights and advocacy. Their work has contributed significantly to reproductive justice movements in Canada, from abortion rights to transgender access and reproductive care. In this section, they share information on how gender-affirming hormones and surgeries might affect some people's fertility, pregnancy, and postpartum experiences. They also discuss the impact of a lack of research in the field and what we can learn from the research that exists.

Here's what we know — and don't know — about the reversible and temporary impacts of gender-affirming hormones on fertility and about the more irreversible and permanent effects.

Puberty Blockers

Puberty blockers (sometimes called puberty inhibitors or hormone blockers) are GnRH analogue/agonist medications that can be used to pause, suppress, or delay puberty. Puberty blockers are typically prescribed to young people between the ages of eight and nineteen, with different organizations and healthcare authorities recommending different lower and upper age limits. Here are some key considerations about puberty blockers and fertility:

1. **Fertility while on puberty blockers.** These medications work by preventing the body from producing certain hormones (namely testosterone, estrogen, and progesterone) that are associated

with puberty, sperm production, ovulation, and menstruation. While taking puberty blockers, the body will temporarily stop producing sperm or eggs. Even if the person on this medication is having the kind of sex that can result in pregnancy, it is very unlikely that pregnancy will occur while on puberty blockers.

2. **Fertility after using puberty blockers.** The effects of puberty blockers on fertility are completely reversible, meaning that when stopped, the body will go through puberty the same way it was going to before the medication was started. Unless the person has underlying fertility issues, sperm production, ovulation, and menstrual cycles will return and fertility will not be impacted.

3. **Transitioning to gender-affirming hormones.** Some people stop taking puberty blockers and immediately start taking gender-affirming hormones like testosterone or estrogen. If this is your plan, see the sections on testosterone and estrogen to understand the impacts of each on your fertility.

Testosterone

Testosterone has well-documented impacts on ovulation and menstruation, with the available literature suggesting that suppression of these physiological functions typically occurs within four to six months, depending on a person's dose and administration method. If you are thinking about taking testosterone or if you are already on it, here's what you need to know:

1. **Testosterone is not a contraceptive.** Even though testosterone use can result in your periods being suppressed, it's not always guaranteed that your ovulation will also be completely suppressed. You can have what's called breakthrough ovulation

— even without a period, you might still release an egg. We know that people can and do get pregnant while on testosterone — especially if they miss a dose, are too late or too early on a dose, change administration methods or decrease their dosage. If you do not want to be pregnant, use a contraceptive even if you are on testosterone.

2. **Pregnancy while on testosterone.** Although testosterone is generally contraindicated during pregnancy (meaning that you shouldn't continue taking testosterone once you become pregnant), the evidence to support this guidance is scant and tenuous (Pfeffer et al. 2023). The empirical research on exposure to testosterone during the perinatal period, including its effects on fetal development, is limited and focuses largely on gestational parents with PCOS and congenital adrenal hyperplasia (both conditions that can result in higher-than-typical testosterone levels among people assigned female at birth). As a result of those higher-than-typical rates of testosterone, the primary concern during pregnancy is about "excess androgen exposure," meaning that fetuses will be exposed to surplus androgen during their development. The range of outcomes *purportedly* associated with excess androgen exposure in utero include urogenital and inter-sex conditions, the development of metabolic dysfunctions later in life (including PCOS), children who espouse non-normative sexual identities (as in kids who end up being gay, lesbian, bisex-ual, queer, etc.), and neurodivergence like autism and attention deficit hyperactivity disorder. That said, it would be misguided and inaccurate to claim that excess androgen *causes* these conditions or outcomes since there are numerous confounding factors — further, having an intersex, disabled, queer and/or

neurodivergent child is, for many, not cause for concern! As an example, PCOS affects one in ten people, and it is the potential for higher testosterone rates among people with PCOS from which the concerns about the impact of androgen excess on fetal development arise. However, we do not routinely place people with PCOS on testosterone blockers when they are pregnant. As such, the potential (and largely understudied) risks associated with excess androgen exposure should be weighed against the impact that stopping testosterone might have on your mental health. It could be that staying on low or micro doses of testosterone during pregnancy could be best for you. There is similarly scant evidence on the effects of testosterone on lactation, although recommendations to stop testosterone while you're nursing are likely based on this same concern about excess androgen exposure.

3. **Pregnancy after testosterone.** People can and do get pregnant after stopping testosterone. When comparing cisgender women who have never taken testosterone with trans people who have and then stopped, research on assisted reproductive technology efficacy shows that these two groups have the same egg quality and quantity (Leung et al. 2019). This means that we can be confident that testosterone does not permanently negatively impact fertility. If you do not have any underlying fertility challenges and depending on your age, you can become pregnant even after taking testosterone for years.

Estrogen

Estrogen has well-documented impacts on sperm production, including decreasing sperm quality, sperm quantity, and sperm health. If you are thinking about starting to take estrogen, or if you are already on estrogen, here's what you need to know: some people can produce sperm after coming off estrogen. However, the amount produced is typically very small, meaning that assisted reproductive technologies may be needed.

We do not have good data on how long someone should be off estrogen before trying to collect sperm, nor good evidence about the rates of sperm production after varying periods of estrogen exposure. In 2023, an advancement was made when a group of researchers reported having recovered viable spermatozoa in nine trans women who had stopped gender-affirming hormones (de Nie et al. 2023). In one case, the sperm was recovered by way of testicular extraction, where sperm is collected directly from the testes through a small incision in the testis, when there was no sperm found in the semen itself. In 55 percent of the individuals, semen quality had decreased. This is nevertheless a promising result, suggesting that infertility following gender-affirming hormone initiation is not guaranteed and that the negative impacts of these hormones on sperm can be reserved. Importantly, De Nie et al. asserted that larger studies are needed to confirm their findings; they also indicate that sperm took many months to recover, may require an invasive procedure to extract, and may be of decreased quality — all of which can have negative physical and psychological impacts. It is therefore recommended that people access fertility preservation, like sperm cryopreservation, prior to starting to take estrogen.

Gender-Affirming Surgeries and Family-Forming Considerations

Are you considering having gender-affirming surgeries and want to know whether and how these will impact your plans to start a family? Here's what we know about gender-affirming surgeries and fertility.

Bottom Surgeries. These are sometimes called lower surgeries, and they involve surgically changing a person's external genitals and internal reproductive organs. If you are thinking about having gender-affirming bottom surgery, here's what you need to know:

1. **Vaginoplasty.** Within the context of gender-affirming care, this is a procedure where a person has a vagina surgically constructed. Vaginoplasty alone does not create the possibility of pregnancy in someone who does not also have a uterus and ovaries. There is some evidence that a particular kind of vaginoplasty, called a Vecchietti-based laparoscopically assisted neovagina, provides the ideal conditions for future uterus transplantation. As medical technologies advance, there may come a time that vaginoplasties and uterine transplants together will create the physiological possibility of pregnancy in people who previously did not have uteruses, ovaries, and vaginas. For now, however, there is no way for a person who was assigned male at birth to become pregnant.

2. **Hysterectomy.** A hysterectomy involves the removal of a person's uterus and perhaps also their cervix, fallopian tubes, and one or both ovaries. If one or both ovaries are retained, a person can still undergo egg retrieval even after a hysterectomy. If both ovaries are removed, a person will no longer produce eggs and as such, no egg retrieval will be possible. Following a hysterectomy, a person will no longer be able to become pregnant.

3. **Phalloplasty.** Within the context of gender-affirming care, this is a procedure where a person has a penis surgically constructed. Phalloplasty alone does not create the possibility of sperm production in someone who does not also have internal reproductive structures like a prostate, seminal vesicles, and glands.

Top Surgeries. These are sometimes called upper surgeries, and they involve surgically changing a person's breasts or chest. If you are thinking about having gender-affirming top surgery, here's what you need to know:

1. **Induced lactation.** All humans can lactate and produce milk using their bodies. Some people may find that they produce insufficient amounts to sustain a neonate or child and may need to supplement using donated milk, formula, or co-feeding with another parent; they may also use medications or supplements to help induce more milk.

2. **Milk supply.** Surgeries that decrease the breast/chest size are likely to reduce the supply of milk. Surgeries that increase or augment the breast/chest are unlikely to impact milk supply, although they may increase incidences of engorgement.

3. **Nerves, ducts, tissues, and nipples.** Depending on the type of surgery a person has and the surgical techniques used, top surgeries might impact the nerves, ducts, tissues, and nipples involved in lactation and nursing. If you are interested in preserving your ability to lactate, surgical approaches where the areola and nipple remain attached, and where the tissue beneath the nipple/areolar region is not removed, may be preferred.

5.
Choosing a Donor

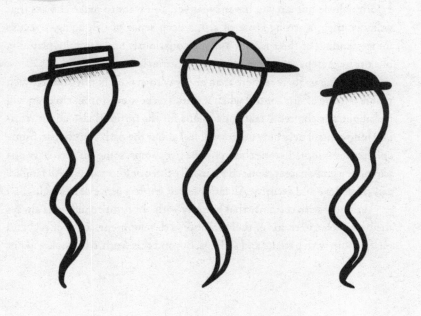

Your decisions are not always linear. You don't need to find your donor before finding a clinic or choosing a method, but each choice will inform the others in different ways. Read this part if you are thinking about using donor gametes (sperm and eggs) and want some guidance navigating your options and preferences. Not all 2SLGBTQ+ families need a donor. Some of us enter the journey knowing what we need. Some of us are surprised to find out what we need. Some of us aren't yet sure what we need. And for some of us, the answer will change.

Picking a donor is a big decision. It can be so hard to imagine what is best for the little human you haven't met yet. You want to make choices that will give them a strong sense of self, a deep sense of belonging, a secure understanding of their family. You are consciously and carefully planning out the next steps and there are so many variables to consider.

The thing is: there is more than one way to make a family and so much that is outside of our control when it comes to how our future children will feel about our choices. Making decisions for the future is also about relinquishing control over how others will feel about the path you choose. Some children are adopted, some children have two moms, some children have one parent or a grandparent, some children have three or four parents. All families can create love and security. All families can create a sense of belonging.

We know with certainty that honesty with our future children is always the best choice in terms of their emotional development, sense of self, and relationship with parents and siblings. Beyond this truth, this book will not privilege any choice over another. Using a bank is a wonderful option for many families and using a known donor is a wonderful option for others. There are choices and conversations to navigate with either option and neither one should be seen as simple or superior.

WHERE TO START

It can be hard to start the process of finding a donor, whether you are planning to use an egg or sperm bank or planning to find a known donor through friends, family, or acquaintances. The first step is thinking through what you want. What is your ideal situation; where are you flexible? What are your must-haves? What kind of medical history do you want to see? What tests do you want a donor to complete? What kind of relationship do you want them (or their family) to have with your family? Will you try to make contact with donor siblings — and how will you feel if your child wants to do so in the future? What are the deal breakers? Try to think long term. Spend time sitting with the what-ifs. Write down your fears, your dreams, your aims, your plans, and your backup plans. Think carefully with your co-parents or partners about what you want before asking someone else to commit. Your clarity is incredibly important in deciding if you want an anonymous, open-ID, or known donor. While we can't predict exactly how our choices for family building will shape our future children, we do know one thing is not debatable: *honesty* is a huge predictor of stability and healthy relationships in all realms. Donor-conceived people consistently emphasize the need for transparency and openness regarding conception and donor choices. Transparency with your future children from an early age can make a huge difference in stability, security, and trust.

In the following sections, I break down some options for egg and sperm donors, ranging from vials purchased from a bank (anonymous or open ID) to known donors and questions to consider when asking community members, family, or friends to be your donor. First, Britt Kernen, a fertility nurse working in Toronto, Canada, offers an overview of current Health Canada regulations and considerations for using donor gametes.

AN INTRODUCTION TO HEALTH CANADA REGULATIONS

by Britt Kernen

Britt Kernen is a fertility nurse in Toronto, Ontario. Their clinic-based work supporting families on their family-building journeys gives them insight into what it is like to try to conceive through ART as 2SLGBTQ+ individuals and families. In this section, they discuss how to navigate Health Canada regulations and some of the basic questions and considerations you can explore in the early stages of your family-building journey.

As a fertility nurse who is also part of the 2SLGTBQ+ community, I have had the honour of being able to help 2SLGTBQ+ people build their families. This has been a wonderfully rewarding experience professionally and personally. My main goal is to ensure that the community is able to make informed decisions and have the proper resources available to them. Through providing fertility care, I have learned how challenging it can be for the community I am a part of to build a family. So much of this work is about sharing knowledge, ideas, and information to help you map your next steps and the way forward in your journey. As a nurse, I work to eliminate the walls that might be in your way, so that the path to your goals is clear.

For 2SLGBTQ+ people there is rarely an "easy" route to family building, whether choosing a surrogate, a known donor, or a donor through a bank. Each route faces its own obstacles. There can be surprises on the journey that you weren't anticipating or choices that you didn't know you would have to make. Sometimes you will be faced with a fertility diagnosis that you didn't know would be an issue. Diagnoses like decreased ovarian reserve or poor sperm quality can be unexpected news for 2SLGBTQ+ people who haven't tried to conceive before. When planning your next steps or when you are faced with these unexpected challenges, my best advice is to lean on your support systems, community, and healthcare professionals for guidance and support.

In the next sections, I will invite you to "Britt's Corner" to share with you some of the knowledge I have gained working in fertility clinics and supporting 2SLGBTQ+ families. To start, I provide some foundational information on Health Canada regulations and what to expect in the early stages of your process, along with suggestions for navigating regulations and medical procedures.

Health Canada Regulations

In 2020 Health Canada created regulations for third-party reproduction cases. These regulations vary depending on whether eggs or sperm are required and if surrogacy is being used. It is important to know that adherence to these regulations is mandatory for clinics, and there isn't much room for flexibility. Sometimes the rules, procedures, or hoops that your clinic is making you jump through are coming from regulations outside of their control.

To better understand the Health Canada regulations, we can break them down into the kinds of services or needs you are seeking from the clinic. Ask yourself:

1. Do you need donor sperm?
2. Do you need donor eggs?
3. Do you need a surrogate?
4. Will you be using gametes (sperm/eggs) from a bank or from someone you know?

Knowing which option is best for you depends on your priorities, values, and outlook, as well as understanding the Health Canada regulations. Each option comes with its own unique journey.

If You Need Donor Sperm

If you choose to work with a bank, the need to coordinate timing with a known donor is alleviated because you can order frozen vials to the clinic as needed, without requiring a donor to undergo testing. However, choosing a donor from a bank still has its obstacles: there are sometimes availability challenges, and costs for vials and samples can be high as well.

For families/individuals in the 2SLGBTQ+ community who require sperm and are using a known donor, the donor will need to do diagnostic testing and Health Canada testing/assessments. This process typically involves doing a semen analysis and an initial infectious disease screening, and undergoing required reproductive and genetic counselling. The donor will also need to complete other screenings, often involving a physical assessment and medical history. Once the donor has been approved, they typically freeze their sample for later use. It is important to know that this testing/screening needs to be completed within a specific timeframe and therefore can be challenging to coordinate.

Choosing a known donor typically requires more effort to coordinate as the intended parent/parents may need time to decide who their donor will be. Timing, testing, and appointments will also depend on both the clinic's and the donor's availability. Cost for this assessment process and treatment varies as well and generally aren't covered by provincial healthcare programs. There is no standard or universal pricing across the country (or within a province). To find out the fees for this donor assessment process I highly recommend checking with the clinic that you are considering working with and reviewing their costs. You should be able to access transparent prices and costs from a clinic, so you can make the choice that is right for you.

The last requirement is a legal agreement between all parties, which of course can take time to finalize and comes with its own fees. Many lawyers will do a short consultation, so that you can determine if you want to work with them.

If using a sperm bank for an open-ID or anonymous donor, then the banks are responsible for complying with these Health Canada regulations and therefore you are not responsible for this step. This option requires less coordination, given that the sperm sample is already available for use/purchase. However, it does mean that you will have to purchase vials from the bank and that you are limited to the vials that are available (and availability does change!). The cost for each vial depends on the bank, and it can be quite costly; in addition, you will have to pay shipping fees (and be aware of shipping times and delays).

There are a few questions that you might consider when using a bank: How many vials should I purchase up front? What is the difference between washed and unwashed sperm? What are my priorities in choosing a donor? What if I can't find a donor that I like? These are all very common questions and although your clinic isn't able to make the decisions for you, they can provide some answers to help guide your decisions.

Washed versus Unwashed Sperm

When you purchase sperm from a bank you have the option to buy "unwashed" or "washed" sperm. Unwashed means that the sperm contains the naturally occurring ejaculate fluids — the vial contains sperm cells along with other cells and fluids. A washed vial means that that everything except the sperm cells has been removed (or washed away). If you purchase unwashed sperm from a sperm bank, your fertility clinic will wash it before an IUI. There is no difference in pregnancy outcomes when you purchase either washed or unwashed sperm.

When does a clinic need to wash the sperm? If sperm enters through the vaginal canal (as is the case with penile-vaginal intercourse or intracervical insemination), the sperm cells swim up to the cervix and leave all of the other cells and fluids behind. Sperm must be washed before IUI because that swimming process does not occur when sperm is placed beyond the cervix, directly into the uterus.

If You Need Donor Eggs

For families and individuals requiring eggs, similar decisions need to be made on whether to use a known donor or an egg bank. If using someone you know, your egg donor would have to do diagnostic testing and proceed with any Health Canada testing/assessments. Diagnostic testing involves assessing ovarian reserve through bloodwork and ultrasound testing, completing any initial infectious disease screening, and then the various Health Canada requirements/screening can also be completed. An egg donor will have to complete some of the Health Canada testing/screening within a specific timeframe of completing their egg donation. A legal agreement will also be required in these cases. Once approved, your donor will have to then proceed with a treatment cycle and egg retrieval. It is a good idea for you to try to get familiar with the process they are going to go through, so that you have an idea of the steps ahead. If using an egg bank, the bank will have done the Health Canada testing. So, similar to a sperm bank, that step is avoided — however, the costs for eggs from a bank can be very high. When choosing a bank, there are normally several purchasing plans available and therefore it is recommended to research the various banks to find a plan that works for you. There are egg banks in Canada and egg banks outside of Canada that are Canadian compliant.

Typically, when using donor eggs, embryos are created either with the intended parent's sperm or sperm from a bank or donor. It is important to know that if the intended parent/parents are the sperm providers and a surrogate is being used in the future, then they will also have to undergo the Health Canada requirements as they would be considered a donor in the context of the regulations.

If Using a Surrogate

Although Health Canada guidelines do not specifically outline any necessary testing for the surrogate, the guidelines outline that if the intended parents are using a surrogate, the embryos being transferred to the surrogate would have had to be created using Health Canada regulations. As mentioned, when using donor eggs, if the intended parents are providing their sperm for the embryo creation, they will have to undergo Health Canada testing as well prior to creating embryos.

Finding a surrogate can take a lot longer than people anticipate — depending on a range of factors, it can be six to eighteen months and at times longer. Due to this unknown length, I often recommend starting the search sooner rather than later.

Paying Out of Pocket

There is typically no funding assistance for known donor assessments or donor samples, and while you cannot pay a surrogate in Canada for their surrogacy, there are high clinic fees for procedures (not covered by government funding) and reimbursements to pay back to the surrogate for their time, travel, and other expenses that may be associated with fertility care, ranging from childcare while they are at appointments to acupuncture to groceries for healthy food. There are some funding options for the treatment cycles (IVF, IUI, etc.), depending on your province. Those who are creating embryos through IVF may be eligible to have some of their costs covered, and some provinces provide a funded cycle for surrogates. Keep in mind that there are typically waitlists for funded IVF cycles. Always check what the waitlist times are for the various clinics you are considering — clinic times range considerably and sometimes even doctors within the clinic will have different waitlist times.

More to Come...

The aim of this section was to help you understand the basics of the Health Canada regulations that every clinic is required to follow. As healthcare professionals we understand that this process may feel long and frustrating, and ultimately our goal is to help make this process as smooth as possible. In the next few sections, I will hop back into the conversation through "Britt's Corner" and provide some suggestions for making your experience a little easier or knowing what to expect.

CHOOSING SPERM AND EGG DONORS

One of the first considerations to think through when you need (or might need) to use a donor is the level of anonymity or involvement you want in an ideal situation. All preferences are first preferences, and part of this process is about considering what happens if you can't access the donor you imagine (because of medical reasons, availability, communication barriers, consent, or other considerations). There are several options to think about, so if you are co-parenting or partner parenting sit down to share your preferences and boundaries. What do you want? What is a definite no-go? What are your priorities? What are your fears?

Options for Sperm Donors

Unknown or anonymous sperm donor. These donors are somewhat less common than open-ID or known donors. For fully anonymous donors, there is no formal way for the intended parents or the offspring to ever find out their identities. The donor has articulated that they do not want contact or communication with future kin. In this case, the bank typically provides some information about the donor's medical history, genetic screening (depending on the bank), and physical characteristics (sometimes accompanied by images or cropped photos). While consumer DNA testing and direct-to-consumer genetic testing can negate donor anonymity, it is important to remember what the donor consented to and what their intentions were at the time of donation.

Open-ID sperm donor: This type of anonymous donor has added the provision that the donor's identity can be disclosed to offspring when they turn eighteen years old. Typically, in these cases the donor-conceived person would be able to request the donor's name and last-known contact information when they turn eighteen. An open-ID donor has consented to this process and articulated that at the time of donation they are open to contact. In these situations, parents cannot request the information on behalf of their child(ren), even in extenuating circumstances. The open-ID arrangement is intended to provide a possibility for future contact between a child and their donor, if both parties are interested.

If you decide you want to use a donor bank, start looking at catalogues, research the clinic's specific parameters and diagnostic tests as well as which banks you can access in Canada. While there are only a handful of banks *in* Canada and limited donors residing here, intended parents can use Canadian-compliant gametes from US banks. "Canadian compliant" means that those vials of sperm meet Health Canada's regulations, which include stipulations in sections of the Assisted Human Reproduction Act (AHRA) and Safety of Sperm and Ova Regulations. These vials can be shipped to Canada. There is typically a filter on a search for a Canadian-specific site that will help you find donor sperm that can be shipped to Canada.

Known sperm donor. This refers to someone whose identity is fully disclosed to intended parents at the time of donation. Often this is a friend, family member, friend of a friend, or someone you sought out for the purposes of donation through your networks. If you think you might need or want to conceive with the help of a clinic, ask your clinic at the outset if they work with known donors (not all clinics do). Every clinic will have different protocols and policies for working with known donors and learning what each clinic will or won't do early in your process will save you time, anxiety, and aggravation.

In Canada, provinces and territories set their own family laws and regulations that impact rights and procedures for known donors and for establishing who the intended parents are. While some provinces require legal steps to identify and define parentage after birth, others (like Ontario) define parentage based on intentions at the time of conception. It is important that you learn about the laws and processes for where you reside, but also for where your donor lives.

In your ongoing communication with a donor, consider setting up time to discuss: 1) the process you are asking them to take part in; 2) what might happen if the first attempts don't work and methods need to change; 3) the future of everyone's relationships, communication practices, and ideal family structures.

Choosing a donor is always an emotional experience. Consider some of these initial questions when thinking about what matters to you and your family if you are choosing sperm from a bank:

- How much genetic testing do you want to do for yourself or for your donor?
- What are your must-haves, the important-but-not-required items, and the definitely-not boundaries?
- All banks are different and offer different levels of information about donor personalities, pictures, and family details or essays. What is important to you?
- Consider what you might do if there are no donors available who fit your criteria — will you wait? Reassess? Contact banks? Look for a known donor?
- CMV status (see the following text box) will be indicated for donors in a bank and might be a consideration if you know you are CMV negative. You should discuss this with your doctor.

What Is CMV?

Cytomegalovirus (CMV) is a very common virus. While many intended parents have already contracted CMV at some point in their life — meaning they have developed natural antibodies — getting a CMV infection for the first time during pregnancy can increase the risk of birth defects. Testing if you are CMV positive or negative and choosing gametes accordingly can help reduce these risks. Ask your healthcare provider to learn more about CMV, pregnancy, and associated risks so that you can make the choice that is right for you.

Options for Egg Donors

There are a number of options for accessing donor eggs in Canada and there is no one universal "best" route for growing your family. Each option below will have different impacts on timelines, costs, legal requirements, current and future relationships with donors, and necessary medical procedures. If you are already working with a clinic, inquire about what kinds of donors and any specific agencies they work with. Not all clinics work with *all* kinds of donors.

Fresh egg donation (through an agency). In Canada, people seeking an egg donor can work with agencies that will help intended parents match with an anonymous or open-ID donor interested in donating eggs by undergoing a cycle of ovarian stimulation and egg retrieval for the intended family. In these processes, fresh retrieved eggs are immediately fertilized with sperm from the intended parent or from a donor's sperm in a laboratory to create embryos, which are either frozen or transferred into the uterus of a surrogate or parent. The level of communication between intended parents and donor and agreements based on anonymity will vary with the preferences of the parents and donor and on agency policies.

Fresh egg donation most often involves an egg donation agency, which coordinates matching, communication, reimbursements, and guidance, as well as a fertility clinic that performs the testing and procedures. While it is illegal to pay a donor, fresh egg donation often incurs higher fees than using an egg bank to purchase frozen vials because the intended parents are responsible for reimbursing expenses for health procedures, testing, and any other expenses the donor incurred related to egg donation or loss of wages.

Frozen eggs (via egg bank). While it is *not* legal to pay donors in Canada, it *is* legal to buy Canadian-compliant frozen eggs from an egg bank. In these cases, a donor has already undergone an egg retrieval and frozen their eggs with a bank. The eggs are cryopreserved and stored until purchased by intended parents. Once purchased, they are shipped to your fertility clinic and can be thawed and fertilized with sperm (from intended parents or donors). Resulting embryos can then be transferred to the uterus of a parent or surrogate. Frozen eggs can provide flexibility because they can be shipped to clinics across the country and may be more readily available. Studies consistently show that while more expensive and often a lengthier matching process, the live-birth outcomes are higher when using fresh versus frozen donor eggs (Setti et al. 2021; Beshar et al. 2021). In the largest study to date, which explored the difference in live birth rates and clinical outcomes between frozen and fresh eggs, notable differences were seen in frozen donor cycles. Most significantly, frozen donor eggs resulted in a decrease in live birth and clinical pregnancy rates, along with an increase in biochemical pregnancy loss (early miscarriage) (Burks et al. 2024). Importantly, frozen eggs are *not the same* as frozen embryos. Burks et al.'s study results do not apply to frozen embryo transfers (which have high success rates).

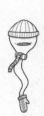

Known donor (fresh or frozen donation). Known egg donation involves using eggs from someone the intended parents directly know (friend, family, acquaintance) who has agreed to undergo the process of egg retrieval for the intended parents. The potential donor will go through initial clinic testing to assess whether they are a good candidate for the process, looking at overall health and fertility, as well as ensuring that they meet any Health Canada regulations. They will then undergo egg stimulation and retrieval at a fertility clinic. Retrieved eggs can be fertilized immediately with sperm from an intended parent or donor and frozen or transferred into the uterus of a surrogate or parent.

Intended parents can opt to work with an external donor agency to manage and coordinate the process (testing, procedures, medications, counselling and legal requirements, and reimbursement), alongside a fertility clinic, which will conduct the testing and procedures. Working with an agency will incur additional fees, but some families choose to do so in order to support and coordinate their process. Not all fertility clinics work with known donors. If this is the method of family building you are hoping to use, it is important to ask a fertility clinic if they offer this service during initial consultations.

Donor Suitability

In Canada, donors (both sperm or egg) must meet safety standards defined by Health Canada and undergo a suitability assessment to evaluate associated risk factors for genetic and infectious disease transmission. A donor suitability assessment involves:

- a physical examination
- donor screening, to collect information about:
  - □ age
  - □ risk factors for particular genetic disease transmission through sperm and egg
  - □ risk factors for particular infectious disease transmission through sperm and egg
- donor testing for infectious diseases:
  - □ HIV
  - □ syphilis
  - □ chlamydia
  - □ gonorrhea
  - □ West Nile virus
  - □ hepatitis B and C

How Many Vials to Purchase

When purchasing vials of donor gametes (egg or sperm), consider your budget and the number of children you want to have. Find out about return policies, refund policies, and availability well in advance of trying to conceive. If using the same donor for all children is important to you, remember that the number of vials available at a bank now may not be available in the future. Vials can be purchased in advance and stored at your clinic or at the donor bank. Thinking about donor availability is important for all methods, but particularly if you are doing IUI since one vial can only be used for a single try. If you are doing IVF, your doctor's goal will be to create as many high-quality embryos as possible so that you can try to conceive multiple times. This means that one vial has the possibility of creating multiple embryos for future use. However, not every egg will result in an embryo and not every embryo will result in a birth. Ultimately, the number of vials you purchase will depend on your budget, the availability of the donor, and your priorities for using the same donor in the future.

Donor Reimbursement and Specific Funding

Neither sperm nor egg donors can be paid in Canada. Instead, we use a model of reimbursing expenses related to donations. If you have a known sperm donor, you are typically paying for any medical expenses (like sperm analysis) and for legal fees and a required counselling session. The process of donating eggs is significantly more invasive, medicalized, and time consuming, and as such the reimbursements are significantly more extensive. Where known sperm donors may need to attend one or two clinic visits to provide a sperm sample, egg donors will need to go through the egg retrieval process, which will require multiple visits for cycle monitoring, testing, and procedures. And in addition to legal, counselling, and medical expenses for procedures and medications, things like wages for missed work due to clinic appointments, childcare while attending the clinic, acupuncture or massage, transportation, and even groceries for healthy food are all eligible for reimbursement.

DONOR EMBRYOS

Embryo donation is a method of family building where individuals or families donate their extra or remaining embryos from completed IVF cycles to those seeking to expand their families. In Canada, fertility clinics typically require an embryo donation agreement before the donation or transfer of embryos can occur. This contract involves embryo donors (those who created the embryos) and embryo recipients (intended parents) and stipulates very clear expectations, agreements, and rights.

The embryo donation agreement addresses parentage, guardianship, future contact, financial support, medical disclosure, and confidentiality. They clearly identify who is and is not a parent, emphasizing that donors have no parental rights and are protected from financial obligations — they are not parents, co-parents, or guardians. Flexibility is allowed in the agreement, customizing it for desired contact between donors and the child, the amount of anonymity desired, as well as potential contact between a donor's children and any children that develop from donated embryos.

Using a donated embryo is a good option for people who do not have their own eggs or sperm to use to create an embryo or viable pregnancy. You can use donor embryos for a pregnancy in your own uterus or with the support of a gestational surrogate to carry the pregnancy. Some clinics have their own embryo donation programs — sometimes referred to as embryo adoption — which allow individuals who have completed their family-building journeys to donate any remaining frozen embryos from their own IVF journey to another person or family. Embryo donation can be done through direct donation (where there is a direct/known recipient or intended parents) or it can be done through closed donation or open-ID donation. If you think this might be a good option for you, speak to your fertility clinic about options available. Even if you are using euploid (genetically tested) embryos, this does not guarantee a live birth. Not all IVF transfers will result in pregnancy and not all pregnancies will result in a baby.

DONOR SIBLINGS ("DIBLINGS")

If you are using a donor, another thing to consider in advance is how you feel about reaching out to those who used the same donor or surrogate. This is possible with any donor (though with a known donor, this is something you can opt to speak openly about with them). Donor-conceived people may choose to use the words "dibling" (donor sibling), brother, sister, half-brother, half-sister, or another term to describe their relations to those who were conceived with the same donor or surrogate.

Scheib and Ruby's 2008 study published in *Fertility and Sterility* looked at contact between families who used the same donors. It found that there were positive outcomes for those who chose to contact each other, and parents typically did so in order to extend family for the child and answer questions about lineage, family, and their donor. Similarly, a 2021 chapter by Vasanti Jadva looked at siblings across families that used diverse mediums for assisted reproduction and found significant variation between what children pursued and how close they were with those who shared a donor or gestational surrogate. Jadva's review of literature found that some children may seek out and form strong bonds with those who were conceived from the same donor or with the same surrogate, but we can't know in advance if people sharing a genetic or gestational connection will form (or be interested in) a sibling-like relationship. While your child will make the choices that are best for them as they grow, parents can make choices around how much contact they want to seek out when their children are young.

There are some formal ways of doing this. Some banks will connect parents through websites or discussion boards, though recently some of these groups have been shut down or discontinued by the banks, so it is worth asking in advance. Many banks also have parent-led Facebook groups where people seek each other out. Donors are identified by their donor IDs and parents can find others who used the same donor for conception. Some parents choose to create chats, groups, or meet-ups for their children and exchange photos or medical information. There are many possibilities and none of them are inherently better or worse. You and your family can decide what is best for you, and it is okay to set boundaries, change your mind, or reassess as you move through your parenting journey.

THEIR DONOR, THEIR LIFE

One hard reality to keep in mind is that the future you envision may not be the future your child ultimately wants. In choosing a donor, think about what tools and strategies you need to develop to cope with change, with differences, and with your future child's choices (which may or may not align with your own). Wanting to find a donor, wanting to remain distant, or perhaps something in between are all options available to your children that do not reflect on you, your parenting, or your successes or failures.

Choosing a donor is not only about having confidence in your own choices, but also about relinquishing control over how your future children will feel about where they came from. We want to imagine a future that is clear, that is predictable, that is *what's best*. And yet, as we build families, each of us must work to remember: we are creating human beings who will have their own journey, their own perspectives, their own questions, and their own hopes and desires. It is so hard for each of us as parents to recognize and sit with what is outside of our control. Because feeling out of control or helpless is hard. It triggers feelings of vulnerability and can make us feel uncertain about the future (because the future is uncertain). We can be sure and confident in our decision and still must be open to our child or children not sharing that same perspective or view.

When we imagine a future family, we can sit with this truth: your baby is a human being who will make choices and have desires outside of your control. What are the strategies and coping mechanisms that you can establish to work through the feelings of vulnerability and helplessness that may arise throughout your parenting journey?

USING A KNOWN DONOR
Communication with a Donor

If you are considering a known donor, it is essential that you have a clear idea of what you are looking for in a donor, both during the family-building process and in the future. Think about immediate needs and future scenarios, including whether extended family will be involved, how any contact and interactions will be managed, and availability for potential siblings. Learn the laws for known donations in your area, as well as the laws where your potential donor lives. You might feel an impulse to rush, but know that the months to find and communicate with your donor are part of the process. Don't jump in without having a clear agreement in place. Three key things to keep in mind as you begin to seek out a known donor and navigate conversations are:

1. **Cast a wide net.** Compile a long list of potential candidates or community members you can reach out to. Be honest if you are reaching out to multiple people at the same time. Your initial email or conversation is not going to have all of the information you need potential donors to know. Rather, think of it as an invitation to engage in further conversations.

2. **Education and information.** Know what you are asking your donor to do. It is important that you understand the basic medical testing or procedures that you are asking your donor to undergo, as well as who they can contact if they have questions (a fertility clinic, doula, physician, or lawyer may be able to provide relevant information). If you can give them a summary and resources and contacts early on in the process, you take some of the guesswork out of their decision making.

3. **Communication.** Know that communication is one of the most important features of a "good" donor. You need to be able to talk to them about your expectations and theirs and to provide boundaries.

The initial contact with a donor is just the beginning of a lifelong conversation between you, your children, and their donor. Even if you do not anticipate any contact or connection with your donor, you need clear communication practices for the initial processes and also the openness and willingness to listen to your future children's desires as they grow.

Making Contact: Initial Letter to Potential Donor

You can choose to ask a potential donor in whatever way works best for you (in person, via phone, or via email). Many people choose to start the conversation through an email or in writing so that the donor does not feel the pressure to immediately respond. Some people choose to send out an email to multiple people at once, while others ask people one at a time. Be transparent if you are asking more than one person.

Below is a sample letter you can revise to send out to potential donors. But the key is to set clear deadlines, give an overview of expectations, and indicate that this is an invitation into a much longer conversation.

Hello [name],

We are writing to a trusted group of friends and family to start the process of trying to make our family. The first thing for you to know is that we won't be offended if you don't respond, and it is okay if you are not interested. We are reaching out to a few different people whom we think highly of to see if they would be interested in potentially donating sperm.

We are emailing you, because we feel our values align and think you would be a great donor. We are not looking for a co-parenting situation. Our donor would not have legal rights or financial responsibilities, but we would like our future children to know who their donor is and possibly have a relationship with them.

We are hoping to move forward with a donor by [INSERT DATE] — but we want to talk more with the donor in detail to come up with a mutually agreeable commitment and plan well before then. Let us know if you have any questions and if you are interested in having a longer conversation about what donating might entail.

Thank you for reading!

Questions for You, Your Co-Parents, and a Potential Known Donor

Before engaging in conversations with potential donors, think through your own preferences for all of the "what-ifs." Questions around relationships, disclosures, even the name you hope that your future children will call the donor are essential conversations to have in advance of donation. But the conversations need to go even further to consider how other family members can or cannot be involved in your initial understanding of and preferences for your family. And what happens in case of illness or even death? What about other children (either the donor's children or other donor families). We need to try to think about every scenario and talk about them, first as intended parents to establish what your family needs and then with potential donors to see if they are a good fit for your family. The tough questions are *tough*. But these foundations are going to be essential not only for these early days of growing your family, but also throughout your family's life, as your child or children grow and as the shape of your family changes. Good communication with *all parents* is essential. If a donor can communicate only with one parent, or if they only find comfort or ease with one parent, this too is in need of discussion and collaboration. The strongest communication practices will lead to the best outcomes for your family.

Once you have initial interest from a potential donor, set up a few times to communicate in more detail. Throughout the next stage of discovery and communication, you can ask your donor the questions listed below and think together about whether or not this person is a good fit for your family-building journey. Give your potential donor time to sit with these questions and reflect on their own boundaries, hard lines, and desires. You are trying to find someone who is the best fit for your family. Listen to your gut, focus on communication, and give everyone time to respond, reflect, and process.

Here are some questions you and your partners or co-parents can pose to a potential donor:

1. Are there any specific medical conditions, allergies, or health concerns that the intended parents should be aware of?

2. Have you done this process before, had any children before, or experienced any losses before? (And do you know what caused the loss?)

3. Has anyone in your family struggled with any fertility issues that you know of?

4. What are your expectations regarding the privacy and confidentiality of the donation process?

5. Are you comfortable with the idea of using a fertility clinic for diagnostic testing and the donation process?
   - For people with eggs, this will entail diagnostic tests, stimulating egg growth, and egg retrieval.
   - For people with sperm, this will entail diagnostic testing, donation at a clinic, or donation at home.
   - For surrogates, this will involve diagnostic testing, embryo transfers, and pregnancy and delivery.

6. How do you feel about the potential travel and time commitment involved in the donation process, including medical appointments and follow-up visits or at-home donation (for sperm) several times a month?

7. Sometimes donations, tests, and procedures cannot be scheduled in advance. The specific date of ovulation can't be predicted. Do you have any travel plans, work commitments, or big events coming up that might be barriers to last-minute requirements?

8.   Sometimes the way we first envision our family-building journey doesn't work out. We might try at home or might try a method at a clinic and realize that it is not working. How do you feel about changing the plan? What process would you want to take if a change in plan was necessary?

Questions about the Intended Relationship

9.   We will need a contract or legal agreement — all fees will be paid by us [intended parents]. Are you willing to sign legal agreements outlining your rights and responsibilities in the process?

10.   How do you envision the child referring to you or addressing you (e.g., donor, uncle, aunt, family friend)?

11.   What are your thoughts on potential visitations with the child? Are you open to periodic meetings or updates? How do you feel about potential involvement in family events or milestones [e.g., birthdays, holidays] as the child grows up?

12.   Do you have any expectations regarding your rights or involvement with the child's life, including decisions about their education, upbringing, or major life events?

13.   If you have children of your own, or if you act as a donor for others, how will we or our child be introduced to them and what relationship to you envision?

14.   What boundaries will exist with your other family members [e.g., donor's family/parents/siblings]? Are you disclosing your donation to them and if so, have you set clear boundaries for their relationship? If you get sick or if you pass away, will expectations or visitations with your family/parents change? How do you envision relationships between the child and your family

members in childhood, adolescence, adulthood — how will you feel if the child requests otherwise?

15. What are your boundaries and expectations regarding sharing the donation process with others, such as friends or family?

16. How do you see your role evolving as the child matures and has questions about their genetic history or donor? What if the boundaries and preferences we set now are different from what this child wants as they grow — how will you react and what modes of communication or relationship building would you want to suggest to them?

Establishing Communication and Relationships

17. What are the best ways for us to communicate with you throughout this process?

18. If we are struggling to communicate or if you are feeling unheard, or vice versa, what is the best way for us to have a conversation?

19. Are you willing to have a conversation with a counsellor or therapist — either together or separately? If we go through a clinic, we are required by Canadian regulations to attend counselling (separately).

20. How can we plan for transparency and openness throughout this process (when we are getting frustrated, when we are reaching a limit, or when we need to set a boundary)?

21. How would you like to handle communication with extended family members or friends who may have questions about the donation process or the child's origins?

READ THIS WHEN

You Are Feeling Good

Right now, you know you got this. Your family will grow, you will be a parent. Your body and mind are capable of this journey. It can be hard to give ourselves permission to just feel good. FEEL GOOD TODAY! You are doing great! Celebrate accomplishments, have a dance party, give a loved one a hug! You deserve this feeling of goodness. Celebrate feeling good!

What is one good thing that happened today?

_____

_____

_____

_____

_____

_____

_____

_____

_____

_____

_____

_____

6.
Choosing a Clinic

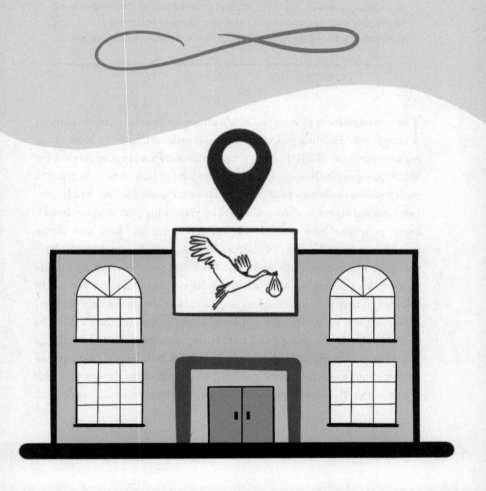

This part is for anyone considering using a clinic for testing, insemination, IVF, RIVF, or surrogacy. There is no "perfect" clinic for everyone, but there may be a clinic that is best (or worst) for you. Advocating for your needs and asking questions can help you feel more educated and empowered in the next steps of your family-building journey. Read this part if you think you might use a clinic or if you don't really know what that entails.

There are a number of ways you might choose to involve a fertility clinic in your family-building process: from diagnostic testing to cycle monitoring to procedures like IUI or IVF, many clinics offer a range of services for 2SLGBTQ+ people. You can choose how much (or how little) you want to incorporate a clinic into your process. There are some barriers and limitations around access to clinics. Geography plays a big part in your choices. Some provinces have multiple clinics, and some just have one. Some provinces in Canada have IVF funding, some do not. Some provinces have year-long waitlists and others do not. So, begin your research by finding local clinics and fertility services. If you have a family doctor, you might ask them if they have any insights, but they aren't always the only (or best) resource. Look for patient-created social media groups for the local clinics or 2SLGBTQ+ family groups and start asking questions. One of the things you may quickly realize is that every experience is different. One person's perfect clinic is another person's red flag, so take all of the experiences with grains of salt. All experiences are valid, but they cannot predict your own.

The point of gathering information is not to make assumptions — it is to learn what kinds of questions are important to you.

You have the right to ask questions.

You get to decide how many questions to ask.

You can always come back to ask more.

Clinics often have good intentions but are overwhelmed or understaffed. This means that emails may go unanswered (even unread) and you may need to follow up. I hope that these next sections help you prepare as best as possible to navigate the ups and downs of communicating with, planning for, and attending a fertility clinic.

WHAT TO EXPECT WHEN CHOOSING A CLINIC

Every clinic is vastly different: how long you wait for your initial appointment, how they communicate with you, who you communicate with, how long you are waiting, and what protocols they suggest. No clinic is the same and each one has both exciting offerings and difficult barriers. Different provinces will have different opportunities and availability for clinic appointments. Some urban centres, like the Greater Toronto Area, may have a dozen fertility clinics to choose from, while entire provinces may only have one (or none!) available. Some clinics may have some provincial funding and others must be paid entirely out of pocket. Some fertility clinics and doctors may require a referral and long wait to even make it through the door, while others can meet

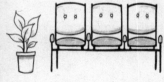 with you almost immediately (mostly those that are paid for out of pocket in urban city centres where there are multiple clinics).

I always tell people that it is not about finding the perfect clinic, but about finding the clinic that works best *for them*. Sometimes this is due to geographical constraints or convenience of location, sometimes it is because of procedures or services that the clinic offers, and sometimes it is because of a shorter waitlist or specific doctor. This is why our family-building journey has to start from us, from our needs, from our priorities, because knowing our priorities will help us to find the clinic that can best meet them. Even though clinics are distinct and the challenges vary, the general process is typically quite standard, especially for people who are pursuing family building for the first time without known fertility issues or barriers. When I try to break it down into what it is *really* like, the truth is that it's surprises, unexpected turns, and often some bumps in the road. Sometimes the surprises are exciting, a second line on the pregnancy stick after one or two tries. Sometimes the surprises are overwhelming, the discovery that your chosen donor cannot take part in the journey, an unexpected test result, a devastating loss. What it is really like are lessons learned, skills gained, emotions and barriers emerging. What it is really like is strategies for navigating communication, roadblocks, and misunderstandings. What it is really like is the biggest joy, excitement, heartbreak, disbelief, and a reorientation of what it means to exist in the world: a new understanding of where we all come from.

The emotional journey accounts for so much. But there are also practical concerns, the day-to-day experience, the expectations for time commitments. So here are some of the basic steps you can anticipate in using a clinic.

GETTING THE CONSULTATION

The first step in introducing a clinic into your process is getting a consultation. It can take months to get an initial appointment, so it is best to move on this before you are ready to start the process of trying to conceive. You can always follow up if you don't hear from the clinic after the anticipated time frame (ask your referring doctor). Some clinics require a referral, so you may need to meet with a GP, walk-in clinic, or sexual health centre for this. Some fertility clinics also have their own affiliated doctors who are able to directly refer you if you don't have access to a doctor. If you are on the fence about using a clinic or don't know if you will need to use one in the future, you can also get on a waitlist or do a consult to collect more information.

If there are many clinics in your area, it can be worthwhile to try to get an initial consultation with a few different clinics to get a sense of the space, prices, priorities, and services offered. For some people, taking the time to meet with multiple clinics can help them to feel in control of their options. If you are struggling to conceive, initial consultations are also good spaces to find out about the range of options available for testing, protocols, procedures, or next steps that they might recommend.

ASKING QUESTIONS AT THE CONSULTATION

Your consultation is a conversation between you, your body, and your healthcare provider to help tailor a starting place for you and a plan that will develop over time. At your consultation, your doctor or nurse will review your test results and medical history. They may ask you some follow-up questions about your lifestyle and habits. But this isn't just a time for them to learn about you, it is also a time for you to learn about them. Taking time during your consultation to ask questions and learn about your treatment options is important. You and your doctor or nurse can discuss timelines, next steps, and ways to best prepare your body to start family-building protocols.

Ask Questions

We can talk about family-building processes and procedures, what to expect from IUI or IVF, how to plan financially, or where to source sperm and eggs, but each of those journeys will be unique to you and your family. One of the hardest parts of family building, especially in the early stages is that *we don't know exactly what to expect* because every journey is different, even for those who have done this before. Each attempt to create a human is a new experience. In order to know what questions to ask a doctor or clinic, we need to have knowledge about processes, expectations, and rights. As you go through each step of your process and learn more information, new questions will arise and old questions will become less relevant. You might choose to ask some of the following questions during a consultation. You can ask all of them, some of them, or none of them. You are in control of your journey.

Potential Questions during Your Consultation

Procedures and Tests

- ☐ What services do you provide (egg preservation, known donor, IUI, IVF)?
- ☐ What initial diagnostic tests do you recommend? If I have had them done elsewhere, can I send you the results?
- ☐ Are there any procedures or tests that have to be done at other clinics, labs, or locations?
- ☐ Can you walk me through the different options we can try (based on my initial test results)? IUI? Medicated timed intercourse? IVF?

☐ What is the wait time for IVF (and if applicable in your province, IVF funding)?

☐ Who performs the procedures at your clinic (doctor, nurses, technicians)?

☐ After I conceive, how long do you continue supporting patients before discharging them? (Some clinics will keep patients in their care for the first trimester while others graduate patients at seven or eight weeks.)

☐ If I experience a miscarriage in my first trimester and surgical intervention is needed, do you perform dilation and curettage (D&C) on site or will you send me to a different clinic?

2SLGBTQ+ Inclusivity

☐ My "legal" name on my health card is different than my name; how will you make sure your technicians, nurses, and other staff call me by the correct name?

☐ Have you worked with trans/non-binary/queer people before? How have your procedures changed to make us feel more included?

☐ I am on gender-affirming hormones, what protocols would you suggest and for how long?

☐ How will you make my partner(s) feel included in this process?

☐ Do you have any 2SLGBTQ+ care advocates, nurses, or third-party coordinators on staff?

Financing and Costs

☐ Can you provide me with a list of basic fees for procedures?

☐ What is the cost structure for fertility treatments, including consultation fees, diagnostic tests, and procedures?

☐ When are payments due?

☐ Are there any financial assistance programs, payment plans, or discounts available to patients?

Treatment Protocols and Timing

- ☐ Can you explain the typical treatment timeline, including initial consultations, testing, treatment cycles, and potential waiting lists?
- ☐ Once my treatment starts, how often will I have appointments, and what is the expected duration of treatment?

Communication

- ☐ How do you communicate with patients (app, phone calls, emails)?
- ☐ If I have questions throughout the process, who can I email or call? What if it is urgent?
- ☐ How often will I speak directly with my doctor?
- ☐ Does your clinic ever "close" (vacation/weekends/stat holidays)? How does that influence scheduling my protocol and treatments?

Other Resources and Supports

- ☐ Do you recommend any supplementary support or therapies (e.g., acupuncture, naturopath, mental health support)?
- ☐ Do you work with specific egg/sperm banks or surrogacy agencies (if applicable)?
- ☐ Are there support groups or mental health practitioners associated with your clinic?

ADVOCACY

We don't always need to know exactly what is happening; we don't need to be doctors, nurses, researchers (though sometimes we do need to learn, to read, to search — everything in moderation). The things you learn in this book or others may not answer all of your questions. This is particularly true for people with medical interventions.

Remember this: You get to press start, stop, and pause. You have a voice in your journey, and you are not alone.

There will almost certainly be moments of confusion, anxiety, and challenges, and it's in those moments that you really need to remind yourself: I have a voice. Put it on a Post-it note on top of your screen, put a reminder in your phone, say it out loud in the mirror. Whatever works! You can ask all of the questions and you can set the pace.

BRITT'S CORNER

• • •

ADVOCATES AND SUPPORT PEOPLE

Unfortunately, it isn't always a linear path when building a family, and there can be unexpected turns. There are counsellors who can provide useful insights and fertility support to both gestational and non-gestational parents.

Whether you are doing this with a partner or on your own, it can be helpful to seek out support for your treatments and perinatal journey. When you go into your cycle-monitoring appointments or procedures, I would recommend having a support person present. If they can't be present in person, see if they can virtually attend via video or phone call during the appointments or if you would be able to debrief with them after appointments.

WAITING

*Trying to conceive is trying to sit with
the unbearable heavy helplessness of waiting.*

We wait for our cycle to begin.

We wait for LH Surge and Ovulation

We wait for Retrieval

We wait for Transfers and Inseminations

We wait for Two Weeks

We wait month after month for a positive test

We wait for the next ultrasound

We wait. We wait.

*The pain and anxiety of waiting animates time.
Our internal clock, our daily activities, our relationships,
and conversations are shaped by the unbearable
weight of waiting.*

*Waiting and sitting with helplessness can trigger intense
emotional responses and insecurities. Know that you
are not alone.*

It is okay to be scared of

what is outside of your control.

FIRST PREFERENCES

Thinking about your first preferences involves thinking about what your ideal path to parenthood looks like and what your next steps will be if you need to shift that plan. It means taking time to consider your priorities, needs, and values. So much of pregnancy, parenting, and family building is outside of our control. There are countless unknowns, changes, surprises, roadblocks, and things rarely go as we first imagine. It is easy to lose track of the things we *can* control: where we start, how we make decisions when things change, and who we invite to the table. Identifying preferences allows you to feel more in control of this process and strategize for care. It provides you with a framework for discussions during a consultation and a better understanding of your own hopes for method, medical intervention, and gametes.

ACTIVITY

• • •

IDENTIFYING FIRST PREFERENCES

Your first preferences are a roadmap for your family-building process. Identify the things that are most important to you, where you want to start, and how you envision this process. Remember that your family's journey is *your* family's journey. Fill out the following worksheet with co-parents, partners, or on your own and identify what your preferences are, where you need to learn more to make a decision, or new questions that come up through this decision-making process. Use this worksheet as a tool for conversation and consideration.

Remind yourself that this is just a starting place. There are many decisions ahead. You are allowed to change and grow.

YOUR FIRST PREFERENCES

This preference sheet is a way to start to think about your priorities, values, and preferences for family building. It is also a way to explore what questions you have not yet considered and what resources would be useful for you.

List three values or positive attributes about yourself that you want to guide your journey and choices.

_____   _____   _____

I hope to use:

☐ My own gametes (sperm or eggs)

☐ A known donor (sperm or eggs)

☐ An unknown donor (sperm or eggs)

☐ An open-ID donor (sperm or eggs)

☐ I'm not sure

I would like to start the process:

☐ At home without medical intervention

☐ At a clinic for basic testing and monitoring

☐ At a clinic with medical intervention

☐ I'm not sure

I would like to start by using:

☐ My uterus

☐ A partner or co-parent's uterus

☐ A known surrogate/friend

☐ A surrogate matched through an agency

☐ Whatever my doctor/provider suggests

I would like to try to family build through (check all that apply):

☐ Unmedicated IUI

☐ Medicated IUI

☐ At-home insemination

☐ Surrogacy with my (or my partner's) gametes

☐ Surrogacy with donor gametes

☐ IVF

☐ RIVF

☐ Penile-vaginal intercourse

☐ I'm not sure

☐ Whatever my doctor recommends

If my preferences can't be met, I would like to...

☐ Continue trying with these preferences for ___ months

☐ Move forward with my doctor's suggested route

☐ Get a second opinion

☐ Press pause until I am ready to try again

☐ I'm not sure

My top four **priorities** for choosing a clinic or provider are:

_____   _____

_____   _____

My biggest **fears** about this process:

_____

_____

_____

_____

_____

_____

My **support network** includes
(add names where it's useful):

- ☐ Partner(s) _____
- ☐ Doctor _____
- ☐ Family _____
- ☐ Friends _____
- ☐ Doula _____
- ☐ Other _____

When I am stressed or anxious, **coping methods** that work for me include:

_____

_____

_____

_____

I would like to find **resources and practitioners** related to:

- ☐ Naturopathy
- ☐ Acupuncture
- ☐ Fertility counselling
- ☐ Relationship counselling
- ☐ Surrogacy agencies
- ☐ Queer community
- ☐ Massage therapy
- ☐ Fertility clinics

One **positive affirmation** or reminder I would like to tell my future self is:

_____

_____

7.
Choosing a Method

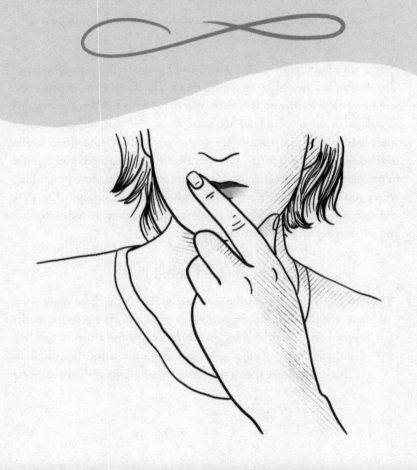

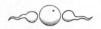

Choosing a method is always about choosing a first method because where we start is often not where we end up. Read this part if you're interested in considering not only the first preference desired by your family, but also to understand alternatives and next steps if you have to shift the processes or protocols you had initially hoped for.

There are a number of ways to try to build your family and a number of environments in which we can do them. The initial choices you make and how you prioritize each of them will shape what options are available to you (what donors you have access to, what clinic you can use (if any), what legal contracts are necessary, where you can try to conceive). The next sections will go through some of the different methods you can use in building your family and considerations for you to explore in deciding where you want to start. Moving from at-home insemination to IUI, IVF, and reciprocal IVF, this overview looks at how to prepare for each cycle and what to expect from the procedures.

HOW TO MAKE A BABY AT HOME

The least expensive and least invasive method for family building is what is often called "at-home insemination" — or, as it is often referred to, the "turkey-baster method" (no, you don't actually use a turkey baster!). Clinically it is sometimes called intracervical insemination (ICI). In this method, the sperm is inserted in the vagina with a needle-less syringe or a non-suctioning menstrual cup. This method has the least medical intervention, as you can do it at home with very few tools. Success rates vary widely based on several factors, such as:

- age of person with eggs/uterus
- quality of sperm
- timing of insemination

Who Can Do At-Home Insemination?

People using a known sperm donor or traditional surrogacy (their egg donor and surrogate are the same person) can do at-home insemination in Canada. You should always have a written agreement well in advance of insemination and know the provincial policies and laws as well as the steps you need to take to ensure clear parental rights.

Additionally, as of 2024, there is *one* distributor in Canada who will deliver sperm vials from a donor bank directly to your home in Canada — allowing people in Canada to use sperm from a bank at home without intervention from a fertility clinic. Through this service, you can order Canadian-compliant sperm and schedule it to arrive during your fertile window (just prior to ovulation, until twenty-four hours after your egg is released). Frozen and thawed sperm has a shorter lifespan than fresh sperm, so timing is even more important.

When you order frozen sperm from a bank to your home, it will be shipped to you in a tank that is charged with liquid nitrogen vapour. The tank can keep the sperm frozen for a few days if it isn't opened. Only open the tank when you are ready to use it, to avoid thawing the sample too early. When your tank arrives, it will have instructions on how to handle the vial and suggested steps for how to do at-home insemination.

When Do You Inseminate?

You are most fertile in the days leading up to ovulation and are no longer fertile twenty-four hours after ovulation. So, it is important to start tracking your cycle before trying to conceive to have a good idea of when you ovulate and how predictable your cycle is. As previously discussed, you might choose to chart your cycle by tracking your BBT, cervical mucus, the position of your cervix, or by using ovulation predictor kits. Some fertility clinics also offer this service (called "cycle monitoring") even if you are inseminating at home.

Once you have signs of ovulation, it is a good time to inseminate at home. Some people choose to inseminate once, while others choose to inseminate two or three times, so that they have a better chance of getting the correct timing. The choice of how many times you inseminate will be informed by how many vials of sperm you have (if you are purchasing banked sperm) or your donor's availability (if you are using a known donor), as well as how confident you are about the timing of your ovulation. There is no perfect formula to predict when you will ovulate in advance of each cycle, so it important to communicate with your donor that there is variability and unpredictability in terms of the ideal timing of insemination each month. You will need them to be available for a few days every month with short notice!

What Materials Are Needed for At-Home Insemination?

+ **Sperm:** obtained from a sperm donor or a partner. It should be collected and inserted as soon as possible. If you need to transport the sperm for any reason, keep it close to your body so that it stays at body temperature.

+ **Sterile container:** for sperm to be collected in.

- **Syringe:** a plastic, needle-less sterile syringe and/or menstrual cup with no suction.

- **Non-suction menstrual cup:** Some people use a cup to hold the sperm close to the cervix after inserting with a syringe; others use the cup instead of a syringe.

What Do I Need to Prepare for At-Home Insemination?

Prior to insemination it is recommended that everyone is tested for STIs and that contracts have been signed to ensure a clear understanding of expectations. Schedule a few months for conversation prior to your first attempt. You don't want this lifelong decision to feel rushed. People can also have sperm analysis done to ensure that sperm are healthy and plentiful.

Finally, if you are using a menstrual cup instead of a syringe to insert the sperm, I recommend practising inserting the cup on its own a few times prior. It's easy to spill the cup and then worry that there isn't enough of the sample left! Try it out a few times before without the sperm so you have a good sense of how to insert it.

INSTRUCTIONS FOR AT-HOME INSEMINATION

1. **Wash hands.** Have everyone wash their hands before beginning to ensure a sterile environment.

2. **Prepare the sperm sample.** If you are using sperm from a bank, follow the instructions from the sperm bank. Ensure you do not open the tank early, or you risk the sperm thawing before you are ready to use it. If you are using a known donor, have the donor either ejaculate into a sterile container or directly into a cervical or menstrual cup. If they ejaculate into a container, load the sperm into the sterile syringe.

3. **Position.** Have the gestational carrier/birthing parent find a comfortable and relaxed position, such as lying down with hips elevated using a pillow and a towel under your bottom. If you are using a cup instead of a syringe, you will likely want to insert it while squatting to avoid spillage.

4. **Insert the sperm.** Gently insert the syringe (or the cup) into the vagina. You can optionally put a menstrual cup in after.

5. **Wait and relax.** You can stay lying down for fifteen to thirty minutes for your own peace of mind (we tend to feel anxious that the sample will "fall out"). There is really not much research to support the idea that raising your hips increases chances of live birth, but it certainly won't hurt to do so for a short period if it makes you more comfortable!

6. **Remove cup.** You can choose to keep the cup in for up to twelve hours (or according to instructions on the box). There may be liquid remaining in the cup — this is normal and does not indicate that the insemination failed or sperm did not travel to your cervix.

What Else Should I Know about At-Home Insemination?

Inseminating at home with a donor or intended parents can look like a lot of different things. In addition to thinking about the steps necessary to help your method succeed, I invite you to think about other elements in the process — emotional, legal, and financial.

If you are using a sperm donor, your method should also consider the legal implications of different methods in different places. For example, in some provinces, the method of conception influences parental rights and assumed parentage. Under BC's Family Law Act, a donor is not a child's legal parent if conceived through ART. However, if a child is conceived through penile-vaginal intercourse, regardless of intention, the individuals who engaged in intercourse are considered the legal parents. Ontario is the only province that recognizes sperm donation through sex, where the donor remains a donor and does not have parental rights. In this case, the parents and donor must have a written agreement in place prior to insemination.

The other consideration that individuals should take very seriously when using a donor in Canada is that you cannot under any circumstances compensate someone for their egg donation, sperm donation, or surrogacy. The consequences for this are *heavy* (ten years' jail time or up to $500,000 fine). There are laws and regulations around how to document reimbursements, so again it is essential that you consult with a lawyer on barriers and policies to expect.

Reading about all of the what-ifs, next steps, best timing, and how-tos can be overwhelming.

Check in with yourself. How are you doing? Are there things in this section that feel good? Scary? Exciting? Confusing? You are not alone in feeling any of these feelings (or all of them at the same time). There are checkboxes and things to do, and then there is also *you*. You and your growing family. Let's tune back into your body and what you hope for its future.

• • •

PUT THE PLAY IN PLAYLIST!

There is so much hardship in this journey and so many barriers. This prompt is to remind you to have fun! Whether this is your first try conceiving or your tenth try conceiving (especially if this is your tenth try!), make time for joy.

Let's make time for a break. Make a playlist of the top ten movies, TV shows, influencers, or songs that bring you joy. After insemination, IUI, transfer, or retrieval, grab a tea or coffee or cookie of your choice and come back here. Take a deep breath, and watch or listen to things that makes you smile:

1. _____
2. _____
3. _____
4. _____
5. _____
6. _____
7. _____
8. _____
9. _____
10. _____

HOW TO MAKE A BABY AT A CLINIC

Going to a clinic is not the same as *choosing* a method. This is because there are different methods and routes you can pursue even if you are going to a clinic: You can consult with a clinic for information to help you determine priorities and best options for your family. You can choose to go to a fertility clinic for basic fertility testing, even if you aren't planning medical intervention and want to try to conceive at home. In some provinces, fertility testing is entirely covered by provincial healthcare, in others some of the tests are covered and not others, and in others there is no coverage at clinics at all. In some provinces and at some clinics, the doctors will help you to track your cycle (using internal ultrasounds and bloodwork) and you can still inseminate at home. In some provinces and clinics, a doctor will prescribe you medication to help in the process of conceiving with a known donor at home. At other clinics, they will only prescribe medication and will only monitor your cycle if you are doing an insemination or IVF at their clinic. This section covers some of the processes and methods that are done at most, but not all, fertility clinics. Key to this journey is *asking questions*. If you are going to a new clinic, ask them what they provide and what they do not do (you can even ask this *before* getting on a consult waitlist — no need to wait for something that doesn't fit your needs!).

CYCLE MONITORING

Cycle monitoring is used at clinics for IUIs, IVF, and timed intercourse (or at-home insemination) to help your clinic track the development and growth of your follicles and the thickness of your endometrium (uterine lining). Cycle monitoring is used for both people producing eggs and gestational carriers to inform the clinic on appropriate protocols and medications and when to schedule an egg retrieval or embryo transfer.

For people who are using their eggs (whether that is you, your partner, or a donor), cycle monitoring begins on the first day of menstruation (day 1). This is when you call or email your clinic and let them know that your cycle has started. They are looking to see how many follicles are maturing and where you are at in your cycle to track when you will ovulate. They will schedule a morning for you to come in, usually between days 2–5 of your cycle. Cycle monitoring usually includes bloodwork and internal ultrasound, followed by information on what medications you should take next.

INTRAUTERINE INSEMINATION (IUI)

Intrauterine insemination (IUI) is a fertility treatment where sperm from a donor or from one of the intended parents is thawed (if frozen), washed, and inserted directly into the uterus. In Canada, most IUI is done at a fertility clinic that specializes in reproductive endocrinology. After your consultation and any necessary diagnostic testing, the process for IUI at a clinic typically involves a few standard steps. Your clinic will have you contact them on day 1 of your cycle so that they can begin monitoring shifts in your hormones and egg growth. If you are doing a medicated cycle, they will prescribe either oral or injectable medications for you to take to stimulate egg growth, usually beginning sometime between days 3 and 7 of your cycle.

With IUI, the aim is to stimulate one to three eggs. In order to reduce the risk of multiples, some clinics will cancel cycles when more than two or three eggs mature. The exact timing and medication will be based on your body and clinic protocols. Once your eggs have matured, the clinic will either trigger ovulation with an injection or allow your body to ovulate naturally and then bring you to the clinic for the IUI procedure. Let's break this down a bit more.

Stimulating and cycle monitoring. During the first two steps you will visit your clinic for cycle monitoring appointments, usually, beginning on days 2–5 of your cycle. Typically, cycle monitoring includes blood-work and an internal ultrasound. If you are doing a natural cycle, you won't be taking medication, but the clinic may do bloodwork and internal ultrasounds to follow your cycle. If you are doing a medicated cycle, clinics may prescribe oral medications (like letrozole or Clomid) or medications (like Gonal-f and Puregon) that are injected daily at home. These medications support your follicle growth. You may also be prescribed a medication that down-regulates the reproductive hormone system (like Cetrotide or Orgalutran). The aim of these medications is to prevent spontaneous and premature ovulation from occurring.

Triggering ovulation. During your cycle monitoring, your clinic is looking at your follicle growth, your lining, and your hormone levels. Once the dominant follicle reaches optimal size (ranging from 16 mm to 22 mm), your lining is thickened, and your body and hormone levels indicate that you are ready to ovulate, your clinic will either schedule your IUI based on your naturally timed ovulation or prescribe a trigger shot to induce ovulation. It is important that you take the trigger shot at the indicated time, because it will be timed with your appointment for your IUI. Timing for your IUI has to be pretty exact, especially if you are using frozen sperm because it has a much shorter lifespan. Most commonly, the trigger shot is administered twenty-four to thirty-six hours prior to the IUI procedure.

IUI procedure. On the day of your IUI, sperm will first be prepared (either thawed by the clinic or donated fresh the day of) and washed. A nurse or doctor will perform the IUI by inserting a speculum to view the cervix and then inserting the prepared sperm into the uterus using a thin and flexible catheter. It usually takes about five to ten minutes. The IUI procedure can feel a lot like a pap smear, which for some people can cause mild discomfort. Following your IUI, you may be prescribed progesterone (which commonly takes the form of suppositories or injections).

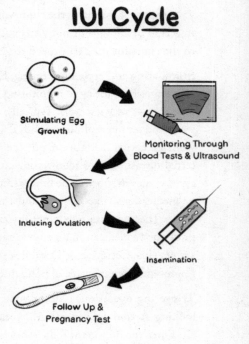

IUI Cycle

Stimulating Egg Growth

Monitoring Through Blood Tests & Ultrasound

Inducing Ovulation

Insemination

Follow Up & Pregnancy Test

What Are the Success Rates?

Success rates for IUI vary *a lot*. Statistics range from 5 percent each cycle to 35 percent each cycle depending on the age of the person with eggs, sperm quality, diagnosis (if any), if you use injectable or oral medications, how many follicles mature during your cycle, and also a good amount of luck. There is higher risk of multiples, especially if you are on injectable medications and mature multiple eggs. Most doctors try to avoid multiples because of the additional medical issues that come with these pregnancies, but there is still a risk. IVF success rates are significantly higher than IUI success rates, but more invasive and expensive.

How Much Does It Cost?

Funding fertility treatments like IUI and IVF is *political* — it changes based on elected officials, party priorities, and policies. Communities across the country have done incredible advocacy to increase funding and access, but no provinces offer fully comprehensive coverage and there are often long waitlists to access funded care, meaning that many families choose to pay out of pocket. While provincial health coverage in some provinces covers the cost of IUI procedures, the majority do not cover medications, the cost of sperm, or clinic-specific service, administration, or washing fees. The exact cost will actually depend on the specific clinic you are working with, as prices are not regulated. Ask your clinic about pricing and ask for a clear and transparent price list of procedures so you know what to expect and can budget appropriately. The current cost of IUI (not including sperm or medications) can range from $400 to $1500 depending on provincial funding for the procedure and clinic fees.

IN VITRO FERTILIZATION (IVF)
What Is IVF?

In its most basic form, in vitro fertilization (IVF) is a process where a person prepares by taking fertility medication (two to three weeks) and then has a procedure done at their clinic (or sometimes a hospital) where eggs are extracted from the ovaries. The procedure generally lasts under thirty minutes. The eggs are then fertilized with sperm outside the body and cultured into embryos. Embryos can then be transferred into the uterus of a gestational parent or surrogate that month, or frozen to be transferred at a later date. We can break it down into a three-step process:

1. stimulating egg growth with medications

2. retrieving eggs for fertilization with sperm in the lab

3. transferring a viable embryo back into the uterus

The experience of IVF can feel more intense than a list of three simple steps. We experience a range of emotions through fertility journeys in part because the process is new and unknown and in part because we feel a lack control over what happens to our bodies and how they might respond. One of the most important things that I remind people who are trying to conceive is not to allow other people's experiences to dominate or limit their own outlook or decision making. Some people have a hard IVF cycle or have side effects from medications, other people have an easier journey. Some people experience big shifts in moods and emotional dysregulation, others feel only a small impact on their mental health and emotional shifts throughout the process. All of these experiences are valid and real, but none of them can predict what yours will be. When we begin the process open to a range of possibilities and experiences, we give our bodies and minds the freedom to experience the process on our own terms.

What Is the Process?

A body typically matures one egg a month naturally, but in order to increase the opportunities for live birth, the first step of IVF is to use medications to stimulate more eggs to develop so that they can be retrieved and fertilized. Through the use of injectable medications, an individual might develop anywhere from one to thirty or more eggs, with the optimal number being somewhere between ten and twenty.

During the process of egg retrieval, mature eggs are fertilized and observed. Any eggs that develop into embryos can be transferred or frozen for future use. In most situations in Canada, a clinic will *only* transfer one embryo at a time to avoid the chance of multiples. While protocols, treatments, and medications will differ based on your body and your needs, the following steps are usually part of the process.

IVF Cycle

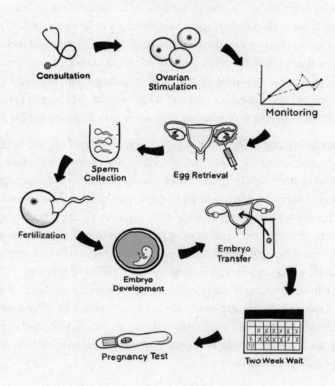

Step 1: "Stimming"

Starting your cycle (day 1). The first official day of your IVF cycle is day 1 of your period. Everyone's body is different, but day 1 is best understood as the first day you bleed (if you have spotting and are unsure, you can always contact cycle monitoring nurses at your clinic). Most clinics will request that you contact cycle monitoring or nurses (by phone, email, or, more recently, clinic apps) on day 1 and the nurses will get back to you within twenty-four to forty-eight hours with a date to come in. Clinics differ in their protocols for how to contact the nurses, when to come in for cycle monitoring, and medications to be prescribed. If you have questions, you can always follow up, ask for information in writing, or if you are at the clinic, you can ask if the nurses are comfortable with you audio recording instructions or taking notes to ensure you understand and remember next steps. You can also ask them to provide an expected overview of what the next few weeks might be like for you.

Stimulating egg growth (days 2–14). Around days 2 to 14, fertility medications, usually hormonal injections, are given to stimulate the ovaries to produce multiple follicles (fluid-filled sacs containing eggs). The goal of this step is to mature multiple eggs that can be retrieved for fertilization. Depending on your age, diagnosis (if any), and ovarian reserve, the expected number of eggs will vary. But if it looks like you will have fewer eggs than anticipated, you can discuss the possibility of cancelling your cycle and trying again with a different protocol.

You start taking these injections daily beginning on day 2 or 3 of your menstrual cycle and continue for ten to twelve days. Everybody is different and the exact timeframe can vary, so your doctor and nurses will check on you at cycle-monitoring appointments to see how you are responding to medications.

In addition to medications that stimulate follicle growth, you may also be put on "antagonists" — medications that will ensure you don't ovulate too early. These medications block the hormone that causes your eggs to be released from your ovaries.

Cycle monitoring. During the time you are stimming, you will be attending cycle-monitoring appointments. These usually consist of an internal ultrasound and bloodwork to watch your follicle growth and hormone levels. This helps the doctors to ensure that you are responding well to the medications and to solidify the timing of your retrieval. Cycle monitoring usually takes place a few times a week and may increase in frequency closer to the retrieval.

Trigger shot. When your hormones are at the right levels and the majority of the eggs are close to maturity (typically 18–22 mm), your clinic will advise you to take your trigger shot at a precise time. The shot will help the eggs go through a final maturation process prior to being retrieved.

Step 2: The Retrieval

The egg retrieval is scheduled for around thirty-six hours after the trigger shot. For some people, the retrieval can feel scary and for others it can feel somewhat routine. It is generally described as causing only moderate discomfort during and following the procedure. Your doctor will help you assess if there are any warning signs to look out for. Everyone's experiences are different. For your retrieval, take the day off of work and plan to have a relaxed afternoon following the procedure. Some people opt to take the following day or two off as well. Listen to your body and your mind and make a plan that works best for you.

Different clinics provide different methods of pain medication and management during the retrieval. Most often the retrieval is performed under sedation (commonly referred to as "conscious sedation"). Depending on the medication used during the procedure and your reaction to it, you may be asleep, drowsy, or completely conscious. During the procedure, using ultrasound guidance, your doctor will insert a needle through your vaginal wall and into your ovaries to collect your follicles. Each follicle is filled with fluid that holds an egg. The retrieval itself usually takes somewhere between fifteen and thirty minutes, depending on how many follicles there are to retrieve.

After your retrieval, in their lab, an embryologist will look at the fluid under a microscope to count the eggs and assess if they are mature. If you are preserving your eggs for the future without fertilizing them, this is the stage when they will freeze them. If you are creating embryos to freeze or transfer, this is the stage when they will attempt to fertilize them.

BRITT'S CORNER

• • •

PREPARING FOR EGG RETRIEVAL

If you have any fears before your egg retrieval or treatment cycle, let your care team know. Letting us know can help us provide more individualized care and be as prepared as possible for your procedure/cycle. You are not a burden. It is okay to ask questions! Our job is to help you during your journey and answer any questions you may have.

From Eggs to Embryos

Typically, your clinic will tell you how many eggs were retrieved immediately following your procedure. The number of eggs they retrieve is not the same as the number of embryos you will have for transfer. You will only know how many embryos you have five or six days after the retrieval, when your clinic will let you know how many blastocysts (or blasts) you have. Blasts are five-day embryos that can be frozen indefinitely. So, what happens to your eggs over those five days? Let's break it down day by day.

Day 0. On retrieval day, your eggs are collected from follicles in your ovaries and the embryologist will determine if they are mature and ready for fertilization.

Day 1. In conventional IVF, eggs and sperm are placed in a controlled environment to allow fertilization to occur. Another method of fertilization is intracytoplasmic sperm injection (ICSI), where a single sperm is injected into each mature egg. Some clinics do ICSI routinely, while others will only do ICSI if there are concerns about the sperm quality. The research is still out on best practice — ICSI is not always shown to result in better outcomes or increased live birth rates. Ask your doctor about what they suggest and why. At many clinics you will get information on how many eggs were fertilized by the end of day 1.

Day 2. Fertilized eggs begin to undergo cell division. You rarely will get an update from your clinic on day 2. Hold tight! Take care of yourself today.

Day 3. Fertilized eggs (also called zygotes) continue to divide and develop into embryos. Usually by the end of day 3, they are at the six-to-eight-cell stage. Many clinics will call you on day 3 to let you know how many day-3 embryos you have.

Day 4. Embryos continue to divide. Typically, clinics do not call to update on day 4.

Day 5 or day 6. This is when many embryos reach the blastocyst stage. The blastocyst has two distinct cell types: the inner cell mass (which will become the fetus) and the outer cell layer (trophectoderm), which will become the placenta. Your clinic will typically inform you of how many embryos you have on day 5 or 6. Blastocysts are then frozen or prepared for transfer at this stage.

Blastocyst Conversion Rates

The more follicles (which contain eggs) you have at the time of retrieval, the better your chances of getting viable embryos to transfer into your uterus. However, the number of eggs you see on an ultrasound prior to retrieval might not be the number of eggs that your doctor is able to retrieve during the procedure or the number of eggs that are mature once observed in a lab. Additionally, not all of the mature eggs retrieved will develop into embryos. This is sometimes called the IVF attrition rate or blastocyst conversion rate. Romanski et al.'s 2022 study looked at how age affects this process. They found that for people under thirty, about 82 percent of the eggs retrieved were mature and had the potential to be fertilized. This rate remained stable until age forty-three. Around 67 percent of the fertilized eggs became blastocyst embryos for those under thirty, and this rate stayed consistent until age forty. However, for those forty-one and older, the rate of blastocyst embryo formation decreased. So, the study indicates that while the number of eggs retrieved might decrease with age, the quality of those eggs, in terms of maturity and fertilization potential, remains steady until a certain age. After that age, the likelihood of embryos forming from fertilized eggs decreases, though it can certainly still occur.

Statistics can only predict so much — every case is different and studies and research rarely make the waiting game any easier for people who are on their family-building journey. You could fall within the statistical likelihood or well outside of it. And that is what makes this all so hard. Waiting for a phone call or email to let you know the status of your egg and embryo development can be incredibly stressful, as we anticipate the number will decrease somewhat with each day. How can you schedule your calendar to avoid big events, work projects, or commitments in the week following your retrieval? What strategies, comforts, or distractions might be useful for you during that five-day period?

Talk to your partner(s) or support people about what might feel good for you during this period. Make a plan for what you can do if the news is not what you want to hear. Do you have someone you can speak with? Do you have ways of giving yourself love and patience over the five days? Thinking in advance about your needs will help you to create a plan for navigating this week.

What do you need and who can you communicate that with? At the end of this part there is an activity focused on communicating needs and sharing strategies for care. Take time to think about what communication means to you before you start the next steps of your journey.

Genetic Screening

If you are doing IVF, you will have the option to do genetic screening on your embryos, called preimplantation genetic testing for aneuploidy

(PGT-A). PGT-A is a screening test done on embryos to identify large chromosomal imbalances or extra or missing chromosomes (called aneuploid embryos). The test cannot create a normal (called euploid) embryo or correct chromosomal abnormalities. Instead, it is a selection tool that might help you decide which embryo to transfer. If an embryo is aneuploidy (or abnormal), your clinic will not transfer it.

If your PGT-A results show different proportions of normal and abnormal cells, this is called a mosaic embryo (or mosaicism). Low-level mosaics have lower percentages of abnormal cells (and higher percentages of normal cells); high-level mosaic embryos have lower percentages of normal cells (and higher abnormal cells). Some mosaic embryos will self-correct as they continue to develop (especially low-level mosaics). If you complete the PGT-A and have mosaic embryos, your clinic will likely invite you to speak with a genetic counsellor to understand your results, the likelihood of successful pregnancy, and next steps. The clinic will have their own internal protocols about how they deal with mosaic embryos and what they are willing or able to transfer. Ask questions about what this means and all of your options.

PGT-A is purchased at an additional fee that is not covered by health insurance (though may be covered by some private fertility benefits). Some clinics charge to test *per embryo*, while others charge one fee for a maximum number of embryos. At some clinics you must decide before your retrieval, while others have flexibility, allowing you to decide post-retrieval. If you are considering PGT-A, ask your clinic about the final deadline to confirm testing.

People who are at high risk of passing on a particular genetic condition can also opt to do preimplantation genetic testing for monogenic disorders (PGT-M), which allows the clinic to look for and identify a specific genetic abnormality or condition. A good example of this is people who carry the BRCA1/2 gene and can opt to test embryos to ensure their children do not inherit it.

There is no right or wrong way approach to creating a family and people can opt to do whatever testing works for them and their family. The important thing to note is that unfortunately, even a euploidy (normal) embryo does not always result in a baby. There are many reasons why I VF transfers fail or miscarriages occur. There is so much that is outside of our control in this process. While testing can give us some information for selecting an embryo to transfer, it cannot determine when pregnancy or live birth will occur.

Step 3: The Transfer

A transfer is when an embryo is transferred into the uterus of a gestational parent or surrogate. It can be done immediately after the embryo develops to the blastocyst stage (called a fresh transfer) or it can be done at a future date, called a frozen embryo transfer. Prior to your transfer, you will discuss how to best prepare your lining and hormones for the process. Preparing your body for your embryo transfer is really about creating the optimal conditions for implantation. Your endometrium is the lining that covers the interior of the uterus and that is where your embryo will implant to achieve pregnancy. There are two key ways of preparing your lining for transfer: a natural cycle or a programmed (or artificial) cycle.

A natural cycle coincides with a biological menstrual cycle. In natural cycles, your transfer will take place following spontaneous ovulation, with minimal medical intervention. These cycles are a bit harder to schedule but allow your body to take the lead and are less expensive. A modified natural cycle is when some medications are used to ensure that ovulation occurs. A programmed or artificial cycle is when medications (estrogen and progesterone) are used to hormonally control and schedule your transfer. These cycles are more predictable but require additional medications. Typically, in a programmed cycle, you aren't ovulating; instead, the medications you are prescribed are creating the optimal environment for your embryo. There has been mixed research on how these two methods impact success, and ultimately it is about what is best for your body, your cycles, and your schedule. It is a good idea to ask your doctor about *both* options to get a sense of which will work better for you and why.

The actual procedure for the transfer is very simple and like an IUI procedure, doesn't require pain medication or sedation. During your transfer, a long, thin catheter containing your embryo is passed through the cervix and into the uterus. The doctor may perform the transfer with or without ultrasound guidance. And then you are done! There is no recovery time from the procedure; you can go home and rest. Take it easy — you did it!

It is important to know that not all transfers will result in a pregnancy. A 2021 study investigating the outcomes of frozen euploid single embryo transfers (FE-SET) found that live birth rates after the first, second, and third transfer were 64.8 percent, 54.4 percent, and 54.1 percent per transfer, respectively (Pirtea et al. 2021). This means that even when an embryo is genetically normal, it may not result in a pregnancy or live birth. Factors that can determine success range from the thickness of endometrial lining, hormones, autoimmune issues, age of the gestational carrier, and just plain old luck.

COMMUNICATION CARDS AND COUPONS

This process is hard and often makes us feel vulnerable. Establishing boundaries, strategies, and practices for care and communication can be essential to helping everyone involved in your journey to feel heard and held. Below are communication cards: copy them, revise them, and change them as needed. They are a starting place to identify what works for you. The idea of the communication card is to have an old-school coupon or IOU to share with a partner or support person when times are tough, communication is hard, and you need something you don't have the words to ask for (let the coupon ask for you). You can have a conversation with your partner(s), co-parents, or support person today to ask how they would feel about using these cards as a mode of communication and if they think it would be a useful way to share needs with each other.

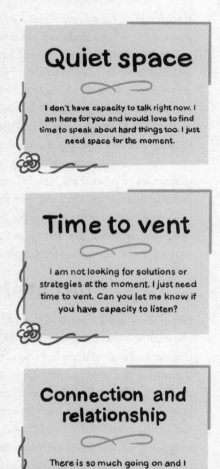

Quiet space

I don't have capacity to talk right now. I am here for you and would love to find time to speak about hard things too. I just need space for the moment.

Time to vent

I am not looking for solutions or strategies at the moment. I just need time to vent. Can you let me know if you have capacity to listen?

Connection and relationship

There is so much going on and I would love a chance to return to "us." I need some time to reconnect.

RECIPROCAL IN VITRO FERTILIZATION (RIVF)

Reciprocal in vitro fertilization (RIVF) is similar to IVF, but in this process one of the intended parents supplies their eggs, fertilized by sperm (donated or from a parent) and a resulting embryo is transferred into another parent's uterus for pregnancy (as a gestational carrier). In this way, two or three parents can be involved in the process of creating and carrying a pregnancy. This is an option for families interested in pursuing IVF who have eggs and uterus in two different parents. The cost for RIVF is typically the same as IVF, but if you have provincial coverage funding your cycle, talk to your clinic about any potential differences in what these benefits cover. When clinics are interpreting provincial coverage, they are not always thinking about the diverse ways in which 2SLGBTQ+ people build their families. There may be some discrepancies, differences, or indeed even confusion when trying to use provincial funding for reciprocal IVF.

PROGESTERONE DURING IVF

Just like we need a medical protocol to prepare the body for an egg retrieval, we also need protocols to prepare the body for an embryo transfer and potential implantation and pregnancy. Part of that equation is ensuring the body has enough progesterone — a hormone naturally produced by the corpus luteum following ovulation. In IVF, progesterone plays an important role in pregnancy outcomes. Progesterone is one of the hormones that can cause physical and emotional shifts in pregnancy, so when you are prescribed progesterone, you might similarly experience some of these pregnancy symptoms even if you are not pregnant. Things like big emotional shifts, fatigue, tender breasts/chest, and bloating are reported side effects. While individuals may experience an increase in new or existing mental health challenges when hormone shifts occur, it is (like too many issues impacting people with a uterus and ovaries) an under-researched area. As Standeven et al. note, "There have been many studies assessing psychiatric symptoms in women undergoing in vitro fertilization (IVF), with variable and overall inconclusive findings. However, there have not been any studies specifically looking at progesterone use in IVF and its effect on mental health" (2020: 117). If you are experiencing mental health shifts at any point in your fertility or pregnancy journey, talk to a counsellor or doctor to work to find a strategy that supports your well-being and care. Sometimes we think we need to "suck it up" or "push through" our pain, as if this is a necessary part of the family-building journey. We minimize our needs because we are afraid they will sabotage our efforts. Working with a provider to support your mental health will not negatively impact your journey to become a parent or to conceive. You deserve to be heard and your experiences (both physical and emotional) matter.

Progesterone Administration

There are various routes of progesterone administration: intramuscular (injection), vaginal or rectal suppository, oral, or gel. Some clinic's standard protocols use one of these routes, while others use a combination. In most cases, you need to stay on progesterone for at least ten weeks (some clinics will routinely keep you on it for twelve weeks), when the placenta will take over its production.

So, which kind of progesterone is right for you? While previous studies and practices favoured intramuscular injections called progesterone in oil (PIO) shots, more recent studies have demonstrated that these difficult-to-administer (and often painful) shots may not offer superior outcomes compared with other routes or combinations. A number of recent studies show no statistical difference in pregnancy or miscarriage rates between those who injected PIO and those who used non-injectable medications (ranging from suppositories to gels, to oral medications, or a combination of these) (Abdelhakim et al. 2020; Xu et al. 2021; Pabuccu et al. 2021).

Other studies have looked at vaginal suppositories *in combination* with intramuscular injections (meaning you may not need to do injections every day) and found this to be just as advantageous as everyday injections (Devine et al. 2021; Jalaliani et al. 2022).

These studies show that PIO may not need to be the first-line standard of care. But, ultimately, there are many factors that will help you and your clinic determine the best protocol for you: the amount of progesterone and how it is administered will depend on your body's needs, your specific protocol, and if you are producing your own progesterone from a corpus luteum (which would be the case if you are doing a natural or modified natural transfer cycle).

How to Inject PIO

If PIO injections are part of your protocol, talk to your nurses about strategies for injection and potential pain management. Administering any injections during IVF or stimming can be really intimidating. Go at your pace and ask questions. There is often a larger needle for retrieving the oil and a slightly smaller needle for injecting. Typically, you will use an eighteen- or twenty-gauge needle to draw the liquid into the syringe, and then switch to a smaller gauge needle (twenty-two or twenty-five) for the actual injection. You can use numbing cream like Emla on your skin prior to injection, if that makes you more comfortable. If you are doing the injection alone, you can also consider purchasing an auto-injector, a device that can help you to self-inject intramuscular medications.

Here are some tips to getting through this hard thing:

+ **Rotate injection sites.** Alternate sides (left and right) and locations (upper outer quadrant of the buttocks) for each injection to prevent discomfort or irritation in one area.

+ **Warm the oil.** Cold oil can be more uncomfortable to inject, so warming it slightly to room temperature by holding the vial in your shirt or hands can help. Do not heat the oil in a microwave or using any other device or instrument.

+ **Remove air bubbles.** After drawing the PIO oil, flick the syringe gently to bring any air bubbles to the top, and then push the plunger to expel the air before injecting.

+ **Relax your muscles.** As much as possible, try not to tense up before the injection. This can help reduce discomfort (sometimes it is easier said than done — exhaling during the injection might help you release tension).

+ **Massage the area.** Gently massage your skin after you inject the PIO to help disperse the oil and reduce the chances of developing lumps where the oil was injected. These lumps are an unavoidable side effect for some bodies. We all react differently and certain methods of injection will be better for some people than others. Massaging the area post-injection and putting warm compresses on the lumps after your injection is one method that helps some people alleviate discomfort and minimize lumps.

+ **Remember that it's different for everyone.** For some people, injections are preferable and easier to manage than suppositories. For others, injections are more challenging. If the method you are using is not working for you, don't hesitate to ask about alternatives or using a combination of PIO and another method, like suppositories.

ABOUT THOSE INJECTIONS

Injections can be challenging, but you might be surprised how quickly you are able to pick up this newfound skill! Doing fertility treatments can make us feel like we suddenly need a medical degree. If you have fears about the injections, let your fertility clinic know, so they can provide more teaching if needed or answer any of your questions. Ask a friend, family member, partner, or co-parent if they can help you. There are also some outside services, like private nurses, that provide injection support, or alternative routes like suppositories that might be available to you.

The best thing to do is to insert the needle as swiftly and firmly as possible! Easier said than done, but if you insert slowly it may hurt more. Some medications cause pain while injecting and this is almost unavoidable. Find the route that works best for you.

THE TWO-WEEK WAIT (TWW)

Regardless of your method of conception or family building, there is no escaping the two-week wait (TWW). The TWW is the period between ovulation and pregnancy test, when you are really in a bit of a limbo — you are hoping for good news, full of anticipation, but this is a vulnerable period given the fear of a negative pregnancy test. Try to talk with your partner or support people before it begins to let them know how you are feeling, what support looks like for you right now, and any accommodations or communication strategies that you are hoping to implement. This is important for *all* partners or intended parents — those who are carrying a pregnancy and those who are not. Make sure everyone involved in your process has an opportunity to share their feelings and needs. The TWW is different for everyone. It may be easy one month and hard the next. It might get easier each try, or it might feel more draining. Every cycle is a new beginning and a new experience. Be generous with yourself and your loved ones.

Another thing you can think about in advance is when you plan to take the first pregnancy test. Individual clinics may differ, but they typically test after about fourteen days for IUI or ten to twelve days post-IVF transfer. They test for pregnancy via blood test and will usually give you a call the day of the test to let you know your result. Some people choose to do at-home pregnancy tests before their blood test. There is nothing wrong with this, but if you took a trigger shot or if you used other medications that contain HCG (human chorionic gonadotropin, the pregnancy hormone) recently, you must be sure enough time has passed for any of these medications to be out of your system. The amount of time it will take for them to leave your system will depend on the dosage (it can take ten to fourteen days).

One thing we often don't talk about is the prevalence of very early miscarriages. If you choose to test early, you may see a line that gets fainter rather than darker. If it continues to fade over a few days, this can be a sign of an early loss called a *chemical pregnancy*. A chemical pregnancy is a miscarriage that happens in the first five weeks of pregnancy, shortly after implantation. Often, this loss occurs without someone even knowing they were pregnant, because bleeding starts around the time of an expected period. If you are testing for pregnancy and there is a faint line with your first morning pee, test again in two days. The line should be getting darker. If the line is getting lighter, this may be a sign of an early loss. While it can be incredibly difficult to grapple with miscarriage at any stage of your journey, it is important to know that in and of itself a chemical pregnancy does not impact your future chances of conception. Once your HCG levels are back to zero, you can try to conceive again, whenever you are ready.

SURROGACY IN CANADA

If you are not able to carry a pregnancy, you can look into surrogacy as an option. There are two kinds of surrogacy in Canada: traditional surrogacy and gestational surrogacy.

Traditional surrogacy. The surrogate carries a pregnancy that uses their own eggs and either a donor or intended parents' sperm — the surrogate is biologically related to the fetus. Importantly, conception cannot occur via sexual intercourse, as assisted reproduction laws do not apply in many provinces to pregnancies resulting from penile-vaginal intercourse. It can be harder to find support (lawyers, clinics, and surrogacy agencies) who will work with traditional surrogacy, out of concerns that the surrogate will change their mind and seek custody.

Gestational surrogacy. The surrogate carries a pregnancy created with either a donor's or intended parent's sperm and eggs — there is no biological connection with the fetus. Gestational surrogacy is significantly more common in Canada because it offers many more legal protections to the intended parents. There has never been a case in Canadian law where a *gestational* surrogate in Canada changed their mind in relinquishing custody of the baby.

How to Emotionally Prepare for Finding a Surrogate

This can be a difficult part of the family-building journey for a lot of people. Not only can it be time consuming and expensive (fees to a surrogacy agency, reimbursements, medical procedures), but it can also be emotionally trying and exhausting. It is important that you are realistic about the amount of time it may take to find a surrogate. For some people, it happens within a few months, but for others the search can take over a year. As you start your process, think about ways to support yourself, strategies for care, and communication and relationship strategies that might be necessary throughout your process.

Who Can Be a Surrogate

Health Canada mandates that a surrogate must be at least twenty-one years old and cannot be paid to act as a surrogate. Fertility clinics (which perform diagnostic tests and fertility treatments) and surrogacy agencies (which match, manage, and coordinate surrogacy arrangements) will also have specific regulations and policies for who they will work with as a surrogate. Many will have a cap on the age of a surrogate, and most will only work with a surrogate who has given birth to at least one child. They will have medical requirements to ensure that the surrogate would be able to carry a pregnancy and is free from transferrable or active STIs. They may also require things indicating a safer environment for a potential pregnancy like requiring that the surrogate doesn't use recreational drugs, will refrain from using alcohol during treatments, doesn't smoke, and lives in a smoke-free household.

How to Find a Surrogate

You can find a surrogate on your own (reach out to your networks, friends of friends, family, community groups — if you are comfortable, get the word out!). Any potential surrogates would work with you and your clinic to determine if they are a good fit and able to carry your pregnancy. You can also find a surrogate through an agency. Surrogacy agencies work to introduce you to potential matches. There are significantly more intended parents than there are available surrogates. So, matching with a surrogate can be emotionally draining — it can feel like you are trying to sell yourself and your family, or trying to prove you deserve this. Let me remind you: *You do deserve this.* Many surrogacy agencies will ask that you create social media posts, videos, or profiles that demonstrate the kind of home you would create, the love of your relationship, and why the surrogate should choose you. This process can feel a lot like jumping up and down and screaming "pick me!" to an audience of strangers. It can be hard, and I wish it were easier.

Surrogacy Agencies

Surrogacy services in Canada walk a fine line. For example, agencies cannot be compensated for directly matching a surrogate and intended parents. They cannot be compensated for managing a surrogate's pregnancy or compensate the surrogate in advance of expenses. They can, however, introduce parents to potential surrogates and have a lawyer privately develop a contract. They can manage clinic services and work to coordinate communication and activities between the intended parents, surrogate, and the fertility clinic that will provide fertility treatments to the surrogate. They can manage and coordinate allowable reimbursements. All of this to say that surrogacy agencies and consulting services can provide some services legally and must abstain from others.

If you are considering working with a surrogacy agency, choosing one to work with is an important step. Use your consultation as an opportunity to gather information about the agency's policies, timelines, and approach. Then be a bit of a detective: after the initial consultation, Google the company, the owners, and community experiences. Via community social media groups, speak with intended parents who've used them. The more information you can gather, the more informed your decision will be. Read their policies carefully. Some surrogacy agencies will have exclusivity clauses or restrictions on your ability to independently find a surrogate at the same time.

Think about a range of experiences, timelines, and services. You might ask questions on:

+ **Timeline.** What is the approximate timeline for finding a surrogate? When will the agency make our profile visible to potential surrogates?

+ **Matching and marketing.** Who will see my profile? Does the agency use social media or suggest the intended parents create posts about their journey? What if we are not comfortable?

+ **Costs.** What costs are incurred for working with the agency?

+ **Surrogates.** How many surrogates does the agency work with and how many intended parents do they work with? How do they screen surrogates and what criteria do they use in their selection process (for intended parents and for surrogates)?

+ **Communication.** Who will be our primary contact at the agency and how often will we receive updates? What modes of communication does the agency use for communicating updates? How do intended parents and surrogates interact?

+ **Fertility clinics.** What clinics does the agency work with?

These initial conversations can feel a bit like talking to a car salesperson: the agency is trying to sell themselves to you and get you on board. Take their answers with a grain of salt and always do follow-up research.

How Are Surrogates Paid?

Surrogates are *not paid*. Only altruistic surrogacy is legal in Canada — meaning people do it out of kindness or a personal drive to do so, not because they are getting compensated. While surrogates are not allowed to be *paid*, they are allowed to be *reimbursed*. Throughout their fertility journey and pregnancy, they must keep all of their receipts for reimbursement. Reimbursement might include the cost of childcare (for their children), medical expenses, travel, lost wages for themselves and for any companion who is with them during appointments.

What Is the Process for Using a Surrogate?

Most surrogacy agencies won't work with you until you already have frozen embryos. Your first step is usually working with a fertility clinic to retrieve eggs from a donor or intended parents and to freeze the embryos.

The typical surrogacy journey looks something like this (if you found a surrogate on your own, the first three points below won't apply):

1. **Creating a profile with the agency.** The profile will usually be distributed to available surrogates online via a website, newsletter, or app.

2. **Meeting potential surrogates.** Once a surrogate selects your profile, you will have the opportunity to view their profile, speak with them and discuss what you are looking for and who you are, and get to know them, their preferences, and if they might be a good match.

3. **Matching with a surrogate.** If you and the potential surrogate meet each other's needs and connect, you will match and move on to diagnostic and psychological testing.

4. **Medical screening and psychological screening.** Surrogates are screened with a basic psychological assessment and fertility diagnostic testing at your fertility clinic.

5. **Legal requirements for both parties.** Your lawyer will prepare a contract with them, discussing all elements of the journey and next steps. Things like fertility and birth preferences, reimbursements for bed rest and lost wages, termination values or protocols for multiples, life insurance for the surrogate, and communication and involvement post-birth are all factors that will be part of your contract conversations. Not all aspects of a legal agreement are enforceable after the contract is signed — for example, the surrogate will always retain the right to terminate a pregnancy and it is their choice to determine who will be their doctor or where they will give birth. But a contract is essential to set out expectations of all parties. It is also important to note that at the time your surrogate gives birth, the location the child is born will dictate some of the legal steps necessary to establish legal parentage. A fertility lawyer can help you prepare for the steps needed to register the birth and ensure that the intended parents take the steps needed to be recognized as legal parents.

6. **Medical protocols.** Fertility protocols can begin after legal contracts are signed. If you are using a traditional surrogate, this will involve going through full IVF or IUI protocol (note: many fertility clinics will not work with traditional surrogacy). If you are doing gestational surrogacy, the fertility clinic will develop a plan and protocol for embryo transfer, including medication to prepare their body for embryo transfer. The surrogate will go to the clinic several times for ultrasounds to look at their uterine lining and blood tests to look at hormone levels. The fertility

clinic will likely have the surrogate start medication a few weeks prior to the transfer and then will perform the transfer — where the embryo is placed in the uterus via a catheter. This procedure is similar to a pap smear.

7. **Pregnancy test.** After two weeks, your surrogate will go into the clinic for an HCG blood test to see if they are pregnant.

READ THIS WHEN

You Are Feeling Tired

Right now, you are exhausted because this process is exhausting. I wish we could skip to the end together and see what happens next. I wish we could rid ourselves of these big feelings easily and just get rest.

What is one way you can care for yourself today?

_____

_____

_____

_____

_____

_____

_____

_____

UNDERSTANDING SURROGACY LAWS IN CANADA

A Conversation with Sara Cohen

> *In this conversation with fertility lawyer Sara Cohen, we discuss the basic legal considerations for surrogacy in Canada. We are really just scratching the surface here, and as Sara says, one of the best places to start is by contacting a lawyer (many give free consultations).*

Laine Halpern Zisman: Can you give an overview of the laws: surrogacy 101?

Sara Cohen: Both federal and provincial laws are applicable to surrogacy. The most consequential federal law is that it's illegal to pay a surrogate in Canada. It's punishable by up to ten years in jail and/or $500,000. Absurd, right? I think the consequence is completely disproportionate to the act, no matter what your perspective is on compensation.

Federal law also stipulates that you have to be at least twenty-one years old to be a surrogate. And with that, you really can't even talk to someone about surrogacy or counsel them about it if they are under twenty-one years of age — it doesn't matter if they are your sister or a relative.

It's also illegal to pay someone to arrange the services of a surrogate or accept compensation for arranging services of a surrogate. And it can be hard to understand this one: What is it "to arrange the services of the surrogate"? Is it to match someone with a surrogate? Is it to arrange their services by organizing their appointments at a clinic, flights, scheduling? We don't have any clear definitions in the legislation.

There is only one case in Canada where someone was charged for paying donors and surrogates and for accepting compensation for "arranging the services of a surrogate." That person pled guilty for paying a donor, but the charges for accepting compensation for arranging the services of a surrogate were all dropped. My best guess is that if someone is helping you choose a surrogate, introducing you to lawyers, helping you get into a clinic, and providing counselling services, etc., then they're not going to be caught by that legislation — but we don't really know because the legislation wording is so vague. We definitely need more clarity, really, on this aspect of the law when the potential penalty is so severe. Health Canada provided clarity for other parts of the AHRA when it set out which categories of expenses are reimbursable. Health Canada does not have the authority to create regulations to explain what it is to accept consideration for arranging the services of a surrogate mother. When something in the law is this vague, it really ought to be struck and the provinces should have the opportunity to regulate instead.

The provincial law, when it comes to surrogacy, is incredibly important because it discusses how parentage is defined and outlines the steps to secure that. The provincial law that applies is in the province *where the baby is born*. In general, you should assume the baby's going to be born in the province where the *surrogate* lives. It's not always that way, particularly where the surrogate lives in a surrogacy-unfriendly jurisdiction such as Quebec, but it is a rare exception when the baby is born in a province other than where the surrogate lives. Intended parents often prefer a surrogate who lives in their province and is close to them, so that they can participate in the pregnancy, but very frequently intended parents and surrogates live in different jurisdictions. As much of Canadian surrogacy is trans-provincial (as well as transnational), it is important to consider this aspect before moving forward with surrogacy.

Every province is different regarding parentage law, the role of intention, and if a formal declaration of parentage process or even adoption process is necessary. In Alberta, for example, in order for the intended parents to be recognized as the legal parents of the baby born through surrogacy, they need one genetic connection between an intended parent and a child. And that's problematic both for practical reasons and because it is discriminatory against non-heteronormative families, as well as heteronormative families who have medical issues where neither parent has viable gametes; not everyone has gametes that are successful in creating an embryo. Additionally, in, Alberta, they don't recognize more than two parents on a birth certificate — whereas in Ontario, for example, you can have four parents on the birth certificate without even seeing a courtroom or requiring any kind of adoption. You just sign the birth certificate with those four names.

In Ontario, Manitoba, and British Columbia, there's no requirement that an intended parent have a genetic connection to the child in order to be parents through surrogacy. Quebec is a whole other story. Until very recently, Quebec law was clear that a surrogacy agreement is void, which made it dangerous for intended parents. Further, without an adoption, it wasn't possible to make an intended mother a parent or to get two dads on the birth certificate. Quebec law is currently changing, but it has some really strict and what seem to me to be impractical requirements. It remains to be seen how the new Quebec law will work regarding the legal parentage of children born through surrogacy.

For everyone, it is really essential that intended parents understand laws across different provinces, not just where they live but also where the baby will or even *may* be born.

LHZ: There are different kinds of surrogacy, as well, in terms of where gametes come from and who will carry the pregnancy. Can you explain the difference between traditional versus gestational surrogacy?

SC: Most of what we see in Canada is gestational surrogacy, meaning that the person who is carrying the fetus is not genetically related to that fetus. This *has* to be done through IVF because the uterus and the eggs are from different people. It can be either a donor egg or the egg of an intended parent and then donor sperm or an intended parent's sperm. Essentially the child is in no way related to the person carrying the baby and the gametes may or may not be related to the parents.

Traditional surrogacy is where there is a genetic connection between the person carrying the baby and the fetus. People might choose to do traditional surrogacy for a number of reasons, whether because it is a less expensive option, it's a surrogate you are really close with, or you want a person's genetics entered into your family — for example, if a gay couple wants a sibling's eggs and uterus to help build their family.

Traditional surrogacy could be done through at-home insemination, and theoretically it can be done through IUI or even through IVF. I say *theoretically* because very few clinics will get involved in traditional surrogacy, for various reasons. Nowhere in Canada is traditional surrogacy recognized if it is through sexual intercourse, even though some jurisdictions, such as Ontario, recognize sperm donation through sexual intercourse.

The concern many people have about traditional surrogacy is that if the surrogate is genetically related to the child, it may be more likely they will want to keep the baby. If this were ever disputed, the concern is that a judge would more likely want to keep the baby with the person who carried the baby, if that person was genetically related. We actually don't have case law where a true surrogate, whether traditional or gestational, has tried to keep a baby. We have cases where it is questionable if they are or are not a surrogate, but not where a traditional surrogate tried to keep that baby. Both gestational and traditional surrogacy are legitimate methods of family building. While there is anxiety around traditional, I don't think that in reality we've seen any more problems with traditional surrogates trying to keep a baby than we have with gestational surrogates.

Interestingly, nowhere in Canadian law differentiates between gestational and traditional surrogacy, nor are these words even used in the law at all. But other countries do make a clearer distinction between the two in their laws. In some US states, for example, the law really protects gestational surrogacy and makes clear that a gestational surrogate has no right to that child. But they leave out traditional surrogacy from that understanding. That said, most of the time when you hear people talk about "surrogacy," they're talking about gestational surrogacy. There are a lot of different iterations, and 2SLGBTQ+ people have different options available.

LHZ: Can you speak a little bit on the question of cost, expenses, and reimbursements?

SC: Surrogacy itself is incredibly expensive. If someone is engaging both an egg donor and a surrogate (gestational surrogacy) in Canada and they were using an agency, etc., it can cost anywhere from C$70,000 to $110,000.

LHZ: Can you an explain where that cost comes from, since you're not allowed to pay a surrogate?

SC: While you can't pay a surrogate, you can reimburse them for their expenses. Health Canada has a "Guidance document: Reimbursement related to Assisted Human Reproduction Regulations" that gives details for section 12 of the AHRA and gives us categories for which expenses are allowed to be reimbursed to the surrogate. This doesn't mean you *have* to reimburse them for all of those things. It's by contract. But it outlines what is a permitted reimbursement.

A lot of the cost is for IVF, and then reimbursing a donor, reimbursing a surrogate, the fees from donor agencies, and surrogacy agencies, legal fees, and counsellors. It's truly expensive.

Typically, by agreement, intended parents are responsible for reimbursing surrogates for any expenses that are incurred due to fertility or pregnancy. If you are engaging with a surrogate in another province, you're flying them in and out, putting them in a hotel where they can be comfortable. Then there are lost wages: what happens if the surrogate is on bed rest and has to miss work, and then during the postpartum period? The intended parents typically become responsible, by contract, for lost income. In recent times surrogates tend to be asking for their lost wages to be reimbursed for about six weeks after a baby's born, which is, in my opinion, legitimate, in order to give them a chance to recuperate from the labour and delivery of the child. I rarely see someone exploiting reimbursements or income lost.

Surrogates don't gain any income from surrogacy, unlike in the United States. So, a surrogate has to be in it for altruistic reasons. Some are surrogates for family or friends. There are a lot of people who are touched by the opportunity to help someone else and they tend to want a relationship with the intended parents. I think it's so beautiful. It's collaborative family building. If it's done properly and respectfully, people often come out of it feeling really fulfilled.

LHZ: So, people are getting reimbursed for their expenses, rather paid up front or in advance. How does that process work?

SC: The requirements are pretty rigid. Surrogates have to submit all receipts and sign a document with every expense reimbursement, essentially stating, "I swear that I only spent this amount of money in relation to surrogacy. I didn't get this money from anywhere else." In and of itself, this isn't a problem, but we do have to think about how much time someone has to invest in the paperwork, how organized one must be to make this happen, and how much up front the surrogate has to pay for related expenses, because they are not entitled to be reimbursed prior to spending.

Consider a surrogate living in London, Ontario, driving into Toronto to go to a clinic. They have to pay for the expenses of that trip up front. *After* the trip, they print a Google Maps route identifying the 195-kilometre trip and get reimbursed for the travel. It requires the surrogate to have access to funds in advance, which isn't possible for everyone. With this in mind, we can see how many surrogates are financially stable, because it's better for everyone if they are, including the surrogate.

LHZ: People often wonder, "Where do I start? Do I start with a clinic, or do I start with an agency, do I start asking friends and family?" Is there one place you would suggest people begin their journey working with a surrogate?

SC: One place I suggest that you might start is with a fertility lawyer, to help you get an idea of your options. Many give free consultations. It's important you start the conversation about surrogacy laws and what is permitted before you start talking to people or trying to get pregnant. Going backwards to fix things is *a lot* more difficult and more expensive than it is to just do it right from the beginning and do it safely. Talking to a lawyer earlier in the process can help you understand the framework before you move forward.

I feel very fortunate to be involved in hundreds and hundreds of surrogacy journeys, probably thousands by now, in Canada. And I really love it. It is one of the most compassionate third-party reproduction options. It's extremely fulfilling emotionally for everyone when done properly.

8.
Loss and Grief

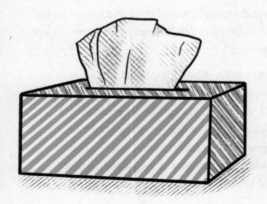

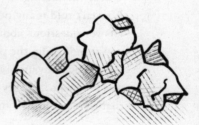

Sometimes we avoid the sad parts, but reading and thinking about loss, and preparing ourselves for the potential of loss can help us imagine what strategies and coping mechanisms resonate with us. It gives us opportunities to share those comfort measures with others. And it allows us to help our future selves through knowledge, curiosity, and communication.

This part is intended to be not only a way to process grief that you've been through, but also to help you to think (and talk) about grief that may come. Learn how to care for yourself and how you want to be cared for by others. Read this part if you are experiencing loss, feeling grief, or trying to conceive, trying to build your family, or thinking about trying to build your family.

One of the hardest realities of queer family building is that we don't get to put oppression on hold. Heterosexism, cissexism, homophobia, and transphobia shape the happy times, the confusing times, and the times of loss and pain. Sometimes it is in these moments of grief that inequities feel most apparent and we feel most alone. Kaley Kennedy (2018) recalls her experience of loss as a queer parent:

> Queer miscarriage comes with other misplaced questions. I haven't told many people [until now] because how do you answer questions about the mechanics of conception when you're mourning the possibility of a different world? While I went about my un-pregnant life, it felt like everyone in my life was pregnant.... Everywhere I went were these swollen bellies that were not misses and not mine.

As queer families, when we grieve and mourn loss, we lose the possibility of living the future we imagined and simultaneously continue to navigate homonormative and cissexist environments and practices. The pain of miscarriage is often exacerbated by a lack of services, support, and resources tailored to our families (Craven and Peel 2017).

I wish there was an easy answer for this. I wish there was a one-stop shop for mourning together, some medium for collectivity and harnessing the knowledge that queer and trans kin are with you, or some tangible reminders that so many of us have been in this space of loss and complete and utterly overwhelming sadness before. There are targeted resources, scattered and sometimes precariously funded, available throughout the country. There are some international services available virtually and a number of in-person support groups and services in provinces across Canada. There are also local therapists who focus on perinatal mental health and queer death and grief doulas whose work specifically focuses on navigating loss and mourning. But these resources come and go because they often lack operational funding, they aren't part of our healthcare system, and the specific needs of minority groups are rarely prioritized. At the end of Part 8, there is a list of websites you can visit with services listed. It is not an exhaustive list, new groups emerge and other groups conclude all the time. Check in with local sexual health clinics, doulas, midwives, or 2SLGBTQ+ social media groups to find available resources.

Ultimately, one of the best ways we can navigate grief and mourning is by building our communities and developing open communication practices. We need to normalize discussions around grief, to think about them in advance, and to build strategies for navigating hard feelings. Loss can be experienced in many ways in this fertility and family-building journey: a failed at-home insemination, IUI, or IVF transfer; the loss of a known donor or the last vial of frozen sperm or eggs; the move from at-home attempts to more medical intervention; embryos that fertilize but don't make it to blastocyst stage; and the loss of a pregnancy through miscarriage or stillbirth. Throughout all of these ups and downs, we are not meant to hold it together at all costs. We are meant to drop and smash and break sometimes. Because this is *hard*. You are allowed to cry, to scream, to be quiet, to be alone, to have sleepless nights. You are allowed to crash and pick yourself back up again or stay low and quiet for the time being.

In this part, I focus primarily on grief and grieving the loss of pregnancy, the rituals we can build to mark times of loss, the conversations we can have even before we start trying to conceive, and the technical and practical considerations if we experience a miscarriage.

Perhaps most importantly throughout this part, I want to remind us: All grief is valid, and all grief has the capacity to change us. It is human to grieve and it is okay for your grief to stay with you for a short time or forever. You do not ever need to forget or "move on." You can sit with this grief in whatever ways feel right for you.

MAKING RITUAL: IT DOESN'T NEED TO BE TIME TO MOVE ON

In moments of shift, moments of pain, moments of wreckage and collapse, we often find that we need *ritual*: an intentional practice to mark a happening, to make us feel held or to hold us when we can no longer hold it together. Sometimes we just need a ritual to guide us with steps for what to do next, so we can go into auto drive and follow a path already paved. Ritual can mark time and make it easier to move through it. But the conventions of time (or how we are supposed to mark and experience time) do not always resonate for people with queer experience. One thing queer theorists and activists have taught us is that queer communities and individual experiences don't easily align with "straight time," or the timelines normalized in white heterosexist Western culture. Straight time tells us we are supposed to grow up, get married, buy a house, have babies, and never ever ever press pause along the way. Productivity, capitalism, a hard rush "forward" are straight time's way of ensuring the past is in the past, the worker is working, the system is profiting. Straight time latches on to the promise of productivity to compel us to leave the past behind and keep on keeping on (Halberstam 2005).

Queer temporality points to feeling strange within the timeline ascribed to you in childhood. It challenges the false notion of a universal desire to follow social scripts. Queer experiences of time, Jack Halberstam asserts, "cannot exist in parallel to a normative heterosexual temporality" (Halberstam in Dinshaw et al. 2007: 182). Queer time reveals the ways in which our normative understandings of power and productivity are based on a timeline that was never meant for us. Queer lives are often not in sync with normative heterosexual existence and *so is queer grief.*

Elizabeth Freeman (2010: xxii) writes that queer temporality's interruptions resist "seamless, unified, and forward moving" time and instead "propose other possibilities for living in relation to indeterminately past, present and future others: that is, of living historically." What a beautiful way to understand our grief and our loss — as our families. We don't need to move forward on an easy-to-follow path.

Queer time allows us to circle back to bring the past into the present, to carry it with us into the future. When we are grieving this can look like destigmatizing remembering, like openly talking about loss. It can mean finding spaces to talk about the future you, the future family, the future baby that are no longer coming. It can mean memorializing the past in the present, creating meal trains (where people send the grieving family food), building rituals, and strengthening chosen family. It can mean valuing the slow pace of grief together, never anticipating a need to forget.

After experiencing a pregnancy loss, some people want to name their baby. Some people want to create a ritual practice to say goodbye, while others want to move to their next cycle without marking the loss. There is no right way to go through grief and sadness. Ritual can mark our experiences in different ways, whether they are rituals at the time of loss, annual milestones or anniversaries to remember, or a photograph, scan, or keepsake, each of these can become tools for sitting with grief and remembering what had been the promise of a future that never came to be. Elizabeth Peel's 2010 survey was the major empirical study on queer women's experiences of pregnancy loss (cited in Craven and Peel 2017). In it, 17 percent of survey respondents had a memorial service, and some of them buried or spread ashes; one had said the Jewish prayer of Kaddish, and some had planted trees or bushes in memory of their child. Some respondents noted that they mark what would have been the child's birthday each year (Craven and Peel 2017). We wear grief on our bodies as it becomes part of who we are, mourning who we thought we would be, and grappling with the changes to who we are. As one of Peel's survey respondents said, "I often feel there should be marks on my body to reflect these pregnancies having happened." We might live in our bodies differently after loss and find new ways to embody it. Miscarriage can sometimes feel like our bodies failed, and coping strategies might look like creating rituals for building new relationships with your physical being. For Kaley Kennedy, this took the shape of a commitment: one hundred swims in one year. Kennedy writes, "It was something to get me through the long days, and the sadness, and the lonely feeling that my body was a mistake....

The effort of my body falls away when I swim. All I think about are the sensations. The feeling of flying. The coolness of water on my skin. My body is working, but it's not labouring. I wish I could experience my body in this way all the time. Only feeling its experiences, and not its effort. I just want it to work, without knowing it's working." Building queer rituals for loss can look like remembering the future you thought you would live and building a relationship with the new person you have become. We can do this all at the same time: bringing the past to the present and into the future together.

PLANNING FOR WHAT WE HOPE WILL NOT BE

We never want to plan for grief. We never want to anticipate the need to mourn, but thinking about your preferences after loss or preparing for the potential of grief can be just as important as the other preparations we go through. At all stages of our family-building journeys, we can normalize conversations about miscarriage, locate supports for loss, communicate our needs and preferences for grieving and rituals, and think about options available for coping with loss and miscarriage (both the practical steps and the emotional needs). If you are building a family with partner(s) or co-parents, or if you have a support person or friend who can support you through your family building journey, set aside time to consider some (or all) of the following questions together.

Grief and Comfort

+ In the past, when we have experienced grief or loss, what has felt most comforting to us (closeness, touch, text messages, in-person conversations, space, alone time, crying together, crying apart)?

+ If we experience a loss, how do we want to refer to the loss or the baby? Do words like "baby," "embryo," or "fetus" resonate most for us right now? Do specific terms or names feel meaningful?

+ Are there particular ways we can think about supporting each other practically (phone calls, meals, planning), emotionally (conversation, space, coping strategies), or physically (touch, proximity, or distance)?

+ Are there rituals or spiritual practices that feel useful in times of grieving?

+ Are there specific ways or significant dates we'd like to mark to remember the miscarriage, baby, or loss?

Communicating with Others

+ How comfortable are we discussing a loss with community members or family? Are there boundaries we want to establish?

+ If we were to experience a loss after announcing a pregnancy, how would we like to handle practical matters such as notifying employers, family members, or friends?

+ Would we be interested in support from a counsellor or group, peer worker, or community leader in helping us navigate a miscarriage?

Self and Community Care

+ What strategies can we develop for dealing with intrusive (or well-meaning) questions from friends or family about our family-building journey?

+ Are there boundaries we need to set on social media or in interacting with community members and relatives who might not be aware of our loss?

+ Are there certain triggers or reminders that we should be aware of in our communication or community spaces? If something is triggering, what do we imagine might feel helpful in those moments (a hand squeeze, leaving the environment, talking about it after the event, moving on without recognition)?

+ How can we ensure that we're taking care of ourselves individually and as a couple while grieving?

+ Do we feel comfortable expressing emotions openly or do we need specific ways to initiate conversations (text message, code word, daily debriefs, couple's counsellor)?

+ How can we balance supporting each other while also taking care of our own emotional well-being?

Future Family Planning

+ How do we want to check in about next steps following a loss?

+ How might loss impact our plans for future attempts at family building?

+ Are there specific steps we want to take to address our emotional well-being before trying again?

+ What steps and strategies can we use if our feelings about next steps don't align? How can we navigate differences, change, or disagreements?

The point of these questions and conversations aren't to devise a definitive guide to grief. The answers to these questions can always change in the future and many of them likely will. The point in initiating the conversation is to start a dialogue and normalize the process of thinking about and valuing our needs. One conversation cannot prepare you for the potential impact of loss and grief, but it can begin the way for ongoing conversations.

IF YOU HAVE EXPERIENCED A MISCARRIAGE

I am sorry you had to say goodbye.

Loss looks like a lot of things — loss does not mean you cannot have family. It may mean you want or need to press pause for a short period. It may mean you want or need to shift your approach or method. Our lives rarely move as seamlessly as we imagine them. In the next few pages, I talk about some of the main questions people who experience miscarriage sometimes ask.

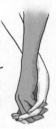

What Is a Miscarriage?

Miscarriage is common. "In Canada, 20–25% of pregnancies end in early or late perinatal death, or about 100,000 deaths for every 376,000 living children" (de Montigny et al. 2018), if we include early losses in this equation, some studies indicate that "50% and 60% of all first-time pregnancies are thought to end in miscarriage" (Annan et al. 2013). The most common reason for a miscarriage is a genetic abnormality. In the vast majority of cases, a miscarriage is not caused by something a parent did. Indeed, in most cases there was nothing that could have been done differently to save a pregnancy. There are different kinds of miscarriage; some of them are what we expect from a loss and others might look a little different.

What Is a Chemical Pregnancy (or Very Early Miscarriage)?

A chemical pregnancy or very early miscarriage occurs during the first five weeks of pregnancy. One of the challenges in finding out you are pregnant very early is that you may also find out you are experiencing an early loss. A person might have a second pink line on a pregnancy test that doesn't progress, or they may have bloodwork done with low or declining HCG levels. A miscarriage at this stage usually is experienced like a heavy period, with variation in how much bleeding there is. The most common cause of a chemical pregnancy is an abnormal embryo. There is typically no intervention needed to complete the miscarriage and typically menstrual cycles return to normal quickly.

What Is Spontaneous Miscarriage?

This is a loss of a pregnancy before the twentieth week of gestation. Spontaneous miscarriages can happen for various reasons, including genetic abnormalities, hormonal imbalances, uterine abnormalities, infections, or other factors. There is often nothing that could have been done to prevent or stop the miscarriage. Symptoms of miscarriage can include vaginal bleeding, cramping, and passing tissue or fluid. According to statistics, 10–20 percent of known pregnancies end in miscarriage, but this number is likely higher. The treatment for miscarriage varies based on if your body has passed all of the tissue (complete miscarriage) or if it needs support to complete this process (incomplete miscarriage) through medication or surgical intervention.

What Is a Missed Miscarriage?

A missed (or silent) miscarriage is when a fetus has passed away and the pregnancy is no longer viable, but the pregnant person's body does not recognize the loss. Like a spontaneous miscarriage, these miscarriages can happen for many reasons (genetic abnormalities, hormonal imbalances, uterine abnormalities, infections, or other factors). The difference here is that the pregnant person may still *feel* pregnant and there are no symptoms of miscarriage like bleeding or cramping. With this kind of miscarriage, some people prefer to wait a few weeks to see if their body releases the pregnancy and tissue on its own, while others use more immediate surgical interventions or oral medications to help their bodies move through the process of releasing the pregnancy and tissue. Think about what you want your next steps to look like and then talk to your doctor about your options. In these conversations, it can be helpful to have a support person with you to help advocate for your preferences, ask questions, or amplify and reiterate your choices.

What Is an Ectopic Pregnancy?

When an embryo implants and begins to develop outside of the uterus, this is called an ectopic pregnancy (or tubal pregnancy, because most often the embryo implants in one of the fallopian tubes). Ectopic pregnancies are never viable. Your fetus cannot continue to grow outside of the uterus. This can also be life threatening to the birthing parent or gestational carrier and medical intervention is needed to avoid a fallopian tube rupturing, severe bleeding, or complications. Different interventions are possible based on your specific circumstances (like oral medications and surgical interventions). The sooner ectopic pregnancies are identified, the sooner the pregnant person is able to receive treatment to ensure their safety. Symptoms can include vaginal bleeding, pelvic pain (often this can happen just on one side), shoulder pain, and weakness or dizziness. You might have all or some of these symptoms. If you experience these symptoms, it is important to reach out to a doctor, your fertility clinic, or a hospital.

How Are Miscarriages Diagnosed?

If you are experiencing a very early loss, your clinic or doctor can do bloodwork to assess your HCG levels. If these are declining or rising too slowly, you may be having a miscarriage. Your clinic will likely repeat the bloodwork to assess if your pregnancy is viable. If you are six weeks or more, your clinic will do an ultrasound to assess the embryo's or fetus's growth and heart rate. Sometimes the results are not conclusive, and you may need to come back for follow up or to assess if the embryo has further developed. Being in this waiting period can be incredibly hard. Be gentle with yourself, find care, and allow yourself permission to feel the emotions that come up here. It can take time to find out if you are losing a pregnancy and additional time for the loss to complete.

MEDICAL PROCEDURES OR TREATMENTS

There are a few different routes for treating early pregnancy loss. You can discuss the best option for you with your clinic or doctor.

1. Watching and waiting (expectant management)
2. Medical management with medications (misoprostol)
3. Surgical management: dilation and curettage (D&C) or manual vacuum aspiration (MVA)

None of these routes is inherently better (or easier), but there may be a choice that is medically and emotionally better for you. Take time to ask questions about the process, the recovery, and what to expect. Finding peer supports who have been through similar experiences can be helpful in understanding the process and feeling a sense of community.

Expectant Management

This approach involves waiting for the body of the pregnant person to naturally pass the pregnancy (sometimes called "products of conception") and is most often an option in early pregnancy loss. It does not require medical intervention, but it can take longer than other options.

When you wait for a miscarriage it can happen immediately or take time to begin. If the waiting period lasts more than two weeks, your clinic or GP may suggest another option (like medical or surgical intervention). According to the Ottawa Fertility Centre, within one week of identifying an early pregnancy loss via ultrasound, one in six people will begin cramping, heavy bleeding, and their uterus will empty. Bleeding similar to a heavy menstrual period can continue for two or more weeks. More than 50 percent of people will experience uterine emptying within two weeks of identifying the loss. Your care provider may monitor you through follow-up appointments, ultrasounds, or bloodwork to ensure that your miscarriage is progressing. If your bleeding stops after two weeks and there are no ongoing symptoms, no ultrasound is needed. Sudden and severe pain, very heavy bleeding (more than three pads in three hours), a fever over 100.4° F (38° C) or sudden dizziness are all signs of an emergency. If you experience any of these symptoms, you should be assessed immediately.

If you ever feel that things are escalating, feeling worse, or you just aren't sure what is normal: check with your doctor. If you feel you are not being heard or taken seriously, or your requests for testing or assessment are being denied, you can: 1) bring a support person to help you ensure your needs are met; 2) request that the refusal to assess or test is written clearly in your charts; and 3) request to speak with a different doctor. You deserve to be heard and taken seriously.

Medical Management

Medical management involve medications such as misoprostol, sometimes taken in combination with mifepristone, taken orally or vaginally to help a miscarriage progress. This medication works by inducing contractions in the uterus that help push the pregnancy tissue from the body. It also causes the cervix to soften. It can be used to *start* the process of releasing the products of conception or to complete the process when the miscarriage has started to progress, but some tissue remains inside the body. The exact dosage may depend on your body and needs. The first does is typically 70 percent effective and the process is up to 85 percent effective after two doses. Symptoms and side effects include bleeding, cramping, diarrhea, and nausea; you may also experience a low-grade fever.

You may start bleeding and cramping as soon as one hour after taking the medication. The bleeding often looks like a heavy period and may contains clots and involve abdominal pain. Prior to taking the medication, ask your doctor, nurse, or clinic who to call in case of emergency or urgent questions. Knowing who to call in advance can help you feel prepared if you have concerns or are experiencing symptoms you weren't expecting. If you do not experience bleeding within twenty-four hours of your first dose, it is important to contact the prescribing physician, clinic, or hospital for next steps. After the initial bleeding and passage of tissue, you will continue to bleed and may experience cramping for up to two weeks. This should decrease with time — if the bleeding remains heavy or if cramping increases, contact your nurse or doctor.

Surgical Management

This is when the contents of the uterus and products of conception are removed through a surgical procedure either at your fertility clinic, an external clinic, or a hospital. This method may be recommended if you have experienced an incomplete miscarriage, if you want a faster method to complete the miscarriage, or for other medical reasons. One procedure often used is called a dilation and curettage (D&C), during which the cervix is dilated and the contents of the uterus are removed via scraping or suctioning. D&Cs can be over 95 percent effective at emptying the uterus. Scraping uses a spoon-shaped tool to manually remove tissue, while suctioning involves a thin tube connected to a pump to gently remove uterine contents with suction. It's a quick outpatient procedure, usually taking ten to fifteen minutes. It is typically conducted during the day, and you will return home later that same day. Following the procedure, you may continue to have menstrual-like bleeding for a week or more. Surgical management results in less bleeding. Speak to your doctor about potential risks, side effects, or other medical considerations.

Products of Conception Testing

If you have had recurrent miscarriages, or want more information on the potential cause of the miscarriage, there may be options, either privately or with your clinic, to test the products of conception, which will look for abnormalities that may have caused your loss. When possible, you need to discuss this option with your clinic *prior* to passing the tissue so that it can be appropriately collected and tested. If you are having your procedure done at an external clinic, confirm with them *before* the procedure that you would like to test the products of conception to ensure that they take the proper steps. This is not a necessary or routine step, but for some people who have repeated losses or who want additional information, it may be a useful tool.

RESOURCES AND SUPPORT GROUPS

There are practical steps and options for treatment, and there are emotional steps and options for support. We need both. Whether you are carrying a baby, mourning a baby, dreaming of a baby who won't come, reach out for peer support on social media, through local queer doulas, or through online groups.

☐ **https://pailnetwork.sunnybrook.ca/**

Pail Network is an online space for loss and grief due to miscarriage or stillbirth. The page has events, support groups (some regionally specific and others based on identity or experience). There is also a page that lists national and provincial resources for loss. Most of their resources and events are not 2SLGBTQ+ specific.

☐ **https://lgbtqreproductiveloss.org**

This is a companion website for the book *Reproductive Losses: Challenges to LGBTQ Family-Making* by Christa Craven. It offers resources specifically for 2SLGBTQ+ families experiencing miscarriage, stillbirth, failed adoption, or infertility. It includes resources for parents, caregivers, friends, family, and medical and mental health professionals.

☐ **https://thelegacyofleo.com/lgbt-baby-loss/**

This is a beautiful website and blog about Leo and the legacy he left behind for his moms. The website has a lot of international resources, stories, and experiences of 2SLGBTQ+ people who experienced miscarriage or stillbirth. The site includes a page of information and resources, most of which are online.

☐ https://pilsc.org/get-support

The Pregnancy & Infant Loss Support Centre is based out of Alberta and serves families internationally. It offers a 2SLGBTQ+ specific support group, as well as peer mentors, resources, and community supports. For families in Alberta, they also offer free comfort boxes.

☐ https://rtzhope.org/lgbtq

This site offers support, resources, and community for people who have experienced loss. While the organization isn't 2LSBGTQ+ specific, one page of their website is dedicated to 2SLGBTQ+ specific resources and information on queer and transgender loss, trauma, and services.

9.
What Is Next?

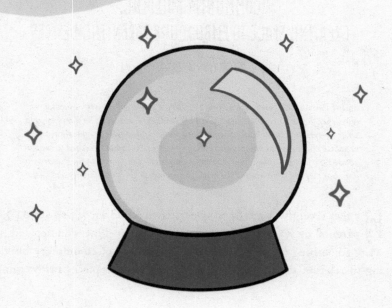

This book doesn't get into pregnancy, labour, or parenting. Instead, it ends by helping to think about shifts and transformations. Our next steps can look like a lot of different things, rarely linear, rarely expected, often weaving in and out, and getting messier than expected. What comes next is tied directly to what came before. This part returns to community building before offering space for transformation and change. Read it if you are navigating transitions and transformations (aren't we all?).

COMMUNITY BUILDING:
CREATING SPACE TO EMBODY OUR PARENTING DESIRES
by *Rachel Epstein and Reese Carr*

Rachel Epstein (she/her) is a longtime 2SLGBTQ+ parenting activist, educator, and researcher. Reese Carr (they/them) is a PhD student, doing work on queer kinship. Their conversation looks back at community resources that were previously available to 2SLGBTQ+ intended parents and looks forward toward what is needed to support 2SLGBTQ+ families today. Their conversation provides insights into the precarity of our resources and supports and the need for ongoing spaces of community and care.

We met recently at a talk on queerspawn (children with 2SLGBTQ+ parents) by Rachel's offspring, Sadie Epstein-Fine, and decided to write something together about the significance of community building in relation to 2SLGBTQ+ parenting. The two pieces below came out of our conversations. At the core of our dialogue was a concern that 2SLGBTQ+ parenting not be confined to a singular blueprint, particularly one that aims to reproduce the hetero-cis-nuclear family. We suggest that living, breathing community spaces, within which people can explore the parenting possibilities open to them, are essential to the growth and expansion of 2SLGBTQ+ families.

Rachel Epstein: In 2001, I was hired as the coordinator of a program called the LGBT Parenting Network, housed then at Family Service Toronto. In 2007, the program became the LGBTQ Parenting Network and moved to the Sherbourne Health Centre in downtown Toronto.

In 2001, I sat at my desk and wondered: how do I start a program for 2SLGBTQ+ parents and prospective parents? As a first step we held a series of focus groups — for longtime lesbian parents, trans parents, gay dads, lesbians considering parenthood, bisexual people considering parenthood, 2SLGBTQ+ stepparents, kids of 2SLGBTQ+ parents, once-married 2SLGBTQ+ parents, gays and lesbians parenting together. All of the focus groups were attended by people with a range of racialized and class identities; we also held a specific group for and facilitated by BIPOC parents and prospective parents.

In the focus groups I asked people about their experiences and about what kinds of programs and resources would be helpful to them. I've summarized their responses as follows:

- We want information and support in order to create families.
- We want connection for ourselves and our children with other LGBTQ+ families, opportunities to hang out, socialize, and talk with others about important issues.
- We are worried about our kids' experiences in schools.
- How do we find queer-positive professionals?

The next fifteen years became about responding to these needs. We developed courses for 2SLGBTQ+ people considering parenthood; discussion series like the Queer Parenting Exchange, where people came together to talk about relevant issues; and social activities and parties for 2SLGBTQ+ led families. We conducted research on adoption, fertility clinics, queerspawn experience in schools, non-biological parenthood — research that produced both academic articles and practical resources and programs. We sat on various government committees and lobbied for policy and legal change to support the recognition of 2SLGBTQ+ parents and families, as well as conducting innumerable workshops and trainings for professionals of all sorts on how to work more effectively with 2SLGBTQ+ families.

Key and central to all of these initiatives was a core commitment to not creating a singular blueprint for 2SLGBTQ+ families — a commitment to recognizing and encouraging expansiveness and creativity in the creation of 2SLGBTQ+ families and offering people an environment in which they could explore and consider a range of parenting options and family configurations. I did not want to fall into "normalizing" 2SLGBTQ+ parenting or attempt to simply recreate the cisgender, heterosexual nuclear family, but to imagine a world in which a huge range of family configurations could exist and be celebrated. A full discussion of the historical and social factors playing into this tension is beyond the scope of this piece, but here I'd like to consider the role that community building plays in the creation of an expansive 2SLGBTQ+ parenting imaginary.

At the heart of the 2SLGBTQ+ parenting programs we created were the family-planning courses, co-sponsored by the Sherbourne Health Centre and the 519 Community Centre: Dykes Planning Tykes; Daddies & Papas 2B; Trans-Masculine People Considering Pregnancy; Queer &

Trans Family Planning. Sometimes run as nine-week, then ten-week, and eventually twelve-week courses, or sometimes over a weekend, we described course goals as follows:

+ Providing practical information
+ Reinforcing a sense of entitlement to be parents (by this we meant understanding the history of oppression and negative ideas about 2SLGBTQ+ parenting, the resulting fears about outcomes for children, support or lack of it from families of origin)
+ Community building

The course facilitators aimed to provide people with practical information about the various routes to parenthood (adoption, conception, surrogacy, co-parenting); to address participants' sometimes buried worries about our entitlement to become parents, often based in societal hetero-cisnormativity and homophobia/biphobia/transphobia; and finally, to build community — to provide opportunities for ongoing connection with others on similar parenting journeys.

While people were grateful for all aspects of the courses (and many, many babies resulted), it was this community-building function that was often the most significant and long-lasting. People formed friendships and support networks through the courses and in some cases continued to meet as a group, or a subgroup, for years afterwards. Their kids knew each other, had play dates and developed their own friendships; these connections combatted the isolation queer and trans parents/families often experience. And, significantly, it was through these community-building initiatives — the panels of 2SLGBTQ+ parents, the panels of queerspawn, the large social and recreational events, the community discussions and celebrations — that people witnessed a range of parenting options, met families of different shapes and sizes and configurations and broadened the possibilities open to them. It was within a living, breathing community that possibilities became realities and imaginations were sparked.

The Sherbourne Health Centre has now shut down the LGBTQ Parenting Network. Since COVID hit in 2020, most in-person programs have gone online. People more and more rely on the internet for information and support. And yet, through my continued work as a fertility counsellor for 2SLGBTQ+ people I am frequently astonished by how many people feel isolated, don't know other queer/trans/non-binary people who are considering parenthood or who have kids, worry about whether their kids will know other kids who live in families like theirs. It saddens me that so many are still grappling with this lack of community. Yes, there are some online support groups — but nothing replaces those in-person, ongoing connections where you and your children can see, touch, feel, and connect with each other. And where, by meeting others, you expand the possibilities open to you.

With the pandemic still raging and social media being the main networking tool, how do 2SLGBTQ+ people with common interests and goals find each other? What do in-person connections provide that virtual relationships do not? Will the lack of in-person connections result in a narrowing of possibilities for prospective 2SLGBTQ+ families? And why are some 2SLGBTQ+ institutions shutting down programs that provide invaluable connections and learning? So much is potentially lost without community support — not the least of which may be continued support for a vast array of family structures and configurations, celebration and expansion of the ways that 2SLGBTQ+ people make family. With fascism and white supremacy on the rise and the human and civil rights of queer and trans people under serious attack, we need each other more than ever — in the flesh. It is through our connections and communities that we can collectively imagine a world that makes space for and celebrates expanded notions of family and of caregiving.

Reese Carr: I am not a parent. I come to think about family and kinship as a young queer person whose childrearing days remain on the horizon. While this is true, I am deeply invested in the possibilities for queer and trans family building that remain open, those that are being foreclosed, and those yet to be imagined. It is through connection and conversation with others, both pragmatic and utopic, that we can envision what we want and need, discover the pathways open to us, and articulate desired pathways that are yet to be created. It is through connections with others in community spaces that information is exchanged, options come into view, and new futures are imagined.

I first became aware of the LGBTQ Parenting Network as an undergraduate student researching queer women's experiences in fertility clinics in London, Ontario. It was while working on this project that I first got a glimpse into expanded notions of reproduction and family in real life, as well as the difficulties that I might experience as a trans non-binary person entering parenthood. For example, despite my inquiries about trans inclusion in the project, the language used of "lesbian, bisexual and queer women" to mean two people with uteruses reflected wider cisnormative ideas about reproduction and family building.

My introduction to the LGBTQ Parenting Network opened up a new and unimagined future for me as I learned about this queer community-oriented program, the reproductive pathways it explored and the parental support groups it offered. The existence of such programs was catalyzed by community members seeking to meet the needs and desires of other community members, and I am grateful for the immense labour, community building and knowledge production carried out at the turn of the twenty-first century by those involved in the lesbian and gay "baby boom." Despite program limitations and room to grow, the existence of the LGBTQ Parenting Network carved out space in the reproductive landscape and provided a push and a model for others.

When I returned to the LGBTQ Parenting Network website a few years later I was saddened to find that it had been taken down; its programs and resources had been relocated within other organizations but then were subsequently shut down altogether. The dreams that I had cultivated were shaken, their foundation cracked. What did it mean that this space dedicated to 2SLGBTQ+ parents and prospective parents, which had been growing and flourishing, no longer existed? While 2SLGBTQ+ community activism has advanced legal and political recognition of a greater range of familial forms, our access to community space remains precarious.

Later in the project, I and the other research assistant attended "Maybe Baby," an information session on queer family planning options in Toronto. It was about a year after I first came across the LGBTQ+ Parenting Network and had started to dream about family-building possibilities. Attending this session and sharing space with other queer people seeking to build families in different ways became a pivotal life moment. Witnessing others carrying out a living, breathing version of something that I had not previously imagined was possible planted in me a seed of curiosity and excitement. In this room, people openly shared their planned family structures, the negotiations that had taken place, and their still unanswered questions. It was here that I first witnessed other trans people taking up parenthood and was able to see myself in these people who were older and in a different stage of their lives. I got to see queer love and desire mixing with the pragmatics of law, policy, and finances. It was in this transformation from the theoretically possible to everyday reality that my vision of what parenthood might look like in my own life started to form.

In thinking about the importance of physical spaces for community building and connection, I am reminded of the significance of interactions that are facilitated through sharing space, like continuing a conversation from a classroom down a hallway and to a café, where friendship is sparked over coffee. These interactions build on one another to create meaningful relationships. Hallways and coffees turn into potlucks, gift exchanges, pet sitting, and food drops through illness.

I did not make connections with the other people in attendance that night, but the in-community visibility had a profound impact. Recognizing myself in others who were living what I hoped for my future brought queer parenting closer to me. Parenting, family, and kinship are fundamentally embodied practices that cannot be reproduced over the internet. While the internet has fostered resource and information sharing for queer and trans people, there are limitations. The internet does not provide hugs after an emotional or vulnerable moment.

For those of us who occupy marginalized identities, the process of becoming a parent can be tedious, emotionally and physically demanding, and, especially for queer people, full of unexpected barriers and roadblocks.

What helps in this process? Information, advice on how to handle the expected and the unexpected, and a sense of community to help breach the loneliness and isolation these processes can elicit. The LGBTQ Parenting Network recognized that 2SLGTBQ+ prospective parents have particular needs that hetero- and cisnormative spaces cannot recognize or meet. The Network provided space to exchange pragmatic information and work for practical, systemic change, as well as to engage in utopic imaginings of our reproductive futures; to interrogate the meaning of "family" while supporting one another's reproductive and parenting journeys.

As we reflected on the changes in queer parenting support in the last few years, it became clear that even as established resources disappeared, people still sought to find and make in-person connections with others entering into queer parenthood. The question for me, then, is why governments, other funding bodies, and the community and health centres that housed these programs were not able or willing to recognize an ongoing need for 2SLGBTQ+ parenting programs and community spaces that facilitate the expansion of community, possibility, and intergenerational connections.

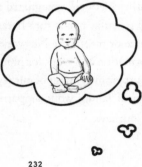

WHAT I WISH I HAD KNOWN

by *Planting the Seed Families*

> When we are trying to build families, our teachers, supports, and advocates are our community members. The people who have been through similar experiences and challenges and can share lived experiences of their journeys. I continue to learn from the remarkable support group participants in the Planting the Seed Fertility and Family Building Group, run out of Birth Mark's Seed and Sprout Program. I have had the true pleasure of facilitating virtual meetings for this group since 2020. This community is composed of 2SLGBTQ+ people at all stages of their family-building journeys, who have advocated for their rights, educated peers, and created and shared resources. They have so much knowledge, experience, and expertise navigating this system. Here they share what they wish they had known about 2SLGBTQ+ family building.

What I wish I had known is how early you would have to make parenting decisions when you are on a queer family-growing journey. There are so many parenting choices you have to make in hypotheticals and before you are even employing bodies to do work in the journey. I think about how all of those micro-parenting decisions require a lot of emotional work and responsibility from you.

There is a lot of grief in a queer family-building journey because our built-in default for a family is heteronormative and so we have to spend most of our existence deconstructing that normative concept, while simultaneously ramping up to make decisions and grow our own families, which is actually really exciting. And if we are not careful and if we don't process the grief of giving up that picture of a family that is ingrained in us, we can pass that shame on to our children. We can put that shame into us at every stage of the journey. Everything that seems "not normal" or takes longer, or seems unorthodox, there starts to be shame attached to it.

I think my partner and I did a lot of emotional work before we got started. I had a lot of grief around the idea of bringing a sperm donor in and having to involve someone else in the process of building our family. But I think letting our grief show, and show large and big and loudly in those early days, made coping when we were (and are) in the thick of the journey easier. It didn't make it happier, but easier. Easier to process our feelings and easier to be confident in the decisions we made and are making.

That is the thing that comes to mind: the pre-processing that is so important. It is an easy journey to throw yourself into because there is so much that you need to do and so much that you need to think about, and nothing really happens quickly. But if I had known that it would pay off later, I would have invested in more emotional processing ahead.

If I was talking to someone now who was just starting out, that is what I would say: check in with yourself emotionally, go to therapy, create a friend group and a community that looks like you, in an intersectional way that is not just queer, but racially, ability-wise, etc. Have those hard conversations. And have them with your partner where you are really processing your *feelings*. Not just your decisions and thoughts. I feel like that will pay off in the future because this is a trying process and going through a process that is so trying requires a high emotional reserve. Processing things ahead of time can help prepare for that.

— Sonya

I wish that I had known that my first plan would also need a second plan and a third plan. I needed multiple versions of a journey that I might be okay with. It took three times as long and had so many more twists and turns than we had ever anticipated. I wish there had been a fairy guide mother who would tell us, "You will get there eventually, but the path will not look at all the way you think it will."

I also wish that someone had told me that I would need to be the advocate for myself, for my community, and for my family, and for my child, and that all of the work and the struggle of trying to navigate a system that is not built for us would, ironically, help me to become an incredible parent and advocate for my child, because that advocacy doesn't stop once they are conceived or once they are born. The struggle we go through creates community and alliances; it makes us the strong, well-informed advocates that our kids need.

— Alison Carson

I wish I knew that when I miscarried, that my mother's response would be "it's because the baby wasn't conceived naturally." That well-meaning straight friends would say "you can still keep trying" after we ran out of embryos, not fathoming that "keep trying" meant finding tens of thousands of dollars again.

I wish I knew that I'd have to become an expert in the law, in medicine, in basic human rights, and make dozens of phone calls and emails before we could even begin to receive equal fertility care as queer people trying to navigate a system not designed for us. I wish I knew that my heart would break a thousand times. For every failed IUI. Every sold-out donor. Every cancelled IVF cycle, every egg that didn't become an embryo, every transfer that didn't take, every baby that grew inside us and whose heart stopped beating. That my heart would stop beating, too, with grief that no straight person could ever feel or understand.

I wish I knew that when my baby finally came, that I'd look at his face every day and wonder if it was really true that he was finally here with us. That the trauma of our journey to parenthood would linger and weave itself into our hearts and make us hold him tight with love and gratitude and unwept tears, and whisper, "you're real, you're here, we made it."

— Ana Luisa Santo

Eight Things I Wish I had Known Navigating Cycle Monitoring and Fertility Clinics:

1. Prepare for wait times at clinic visits. You could be there for two hours or more.

2. Bring a book, music, or a quiet activity to your appointments.

3. Pack a snack or breakfast.

4. Remember, it's a journey, be present in the journey. This is a roller coaster ride!

5. Be kind to yourself. Take the day off after any procedure, not just for your body, but for your mind.

6. When close friends ask what you need, ask for meals.

7. Advocate for yourself. They give general ideas and directions but think of them as educated suggestions. They are providing options; that doesn't mean you have to follow what they say.

8. Find a support group that you feel comfortable joining. It's really hard to go through this on your own. You are not alone.

— Samantha Wynter

We wish we'd known how difficult public adoption is — it is highly dependent on what region you are living in and what is available to you in terms of prospective adoptees. Being in Waterloo Region, we had quite a difficult time getting information and understanding the process. It was a challenge that turned us off and the private sector was way too costly. Fostership takes a lot more than what we could have managed at the time, especially when the fosters are young. The adoption system is something we wish we had known because it was our first choice.

I wish I knew I could say "no" to certain diagnostic procedures. Now that I have given birth, I can say that for me a sonohysterogram was worse. Birth was hard, but at least I was able to manage it with sound and movement and all of the things that help you to function through the process, having lots of supports around me and a birthing pool and all of things that I needed. But that sonohysterogram — if I never have to do another one in my life, I will be thankful!

— Kia

I wish I knew how much misinformation prevails with little to no way to confirm the true experiences. There is an overwhelming amount of information out there and yet there is no information available. The fear of sharing true experiences by the already vulnerable intended parents leaves even fewer reliable sources for the ones just starting on this journey. I wish I knew the true gravity of this journey and also how extremely important support is through it all. Another important thing I wish I knew was how vulnerable this entire journey would be. We literally had to let all our walls down and present our vulnerable selves to the world and it was not easy, not then, not now.

— Ripun

We started our family-building journey with a ton of hope and little information. We were surprised to learn that in Canada, you can't have sperm shipped to your house like you can in the States. For us, as a two-woman couple, our options were to try at home with a known donor or go the hyper-medicalized, fertility clinic route. The surprises didn't stop there — lack of consideration for queer families at the clinic, extra hurdles like mandatory therapy (only for queer couples), the increased isolation of trying to get pregnant during the COVID-19 pandemic, and thinking IVF was a golden ticket to our dream of having a child — it was not. The path we took was winding, devastating, and now I know that it all added up to knowing our perfect daughter, Effie.

In our case, our family-building journey meant that our family expanded beyond welcoming sweet Effie. We often reflect on how the journey to knowing her gave us a deep appreciation for the privilege that it is to be her parents. There's something so unique and precious about the children of queer parents. Our children are dreamed of and fought for — our own understanding of family reimagined in a beautiful way. I hope that family-building journeys will be less traumatic for Canadian queer parents to come. I wish when we were in the thick of it, I had known that I would find peace and appreciation for our journey, and that our experiences helped to prepare us to parent in a heteronormative world.

— Carly Pettinger

I wish I had known that all of the pain to get here... would be so worth it.

You Are Looking for Community

This journey can be lonely. Our histories have been silenced and closeted for so long and our narratives are shared in hushed voices or closed-door rooms. Too often we are made to believe that our history is short or that our stories are new. But our families have always existed. You are part of a history of love and kinship where families are made and supported in all kinds of ways. You are part of long line of Two-Spirit, transgender, dyke, pan, queer, gay, lesbian, non-binary, and gender-diverse peoples. You will raise a family of resistance and love that can create real and lasting change. Find community, build friendships; you are expanding goodness.

What kind of community do you dream of for yourself and your family?

_____

_____

_____

_____

_____

_____

_____

_____

TRANSFORMATIONS:
WHO WE WERE AND WHO WE ARE BECOMING

This is the end of the book, *technically*. These are the last pages, but it doesn't mean it ends here. There are many books on my bookshelf that I come back to time and again. I hope this can be one of those books for you. Come back here for affirmations and reflections. Come back here when things go off course and you need to find a way to navigate new choices. Come back here when you don't know what questions to ask. Mostly, come back here when you feel alone. Sometimes we just need a reminder of the elders and ancestors who have come before us. So much of this journey is about the community, the village, the histories that have laid the foundations for our advocacy, efforts, and families.

I am indebted to the incredible Seed and Sprout community at Birth Mark in Toronto. We have been meeting each month for a few years. Everyone comes to the group with their own experiences, their own stressors, at a different place in their own story in the making. Recently, a new member joined. They were just at the beginning of their journey, trying to find somewhere to ask all of their questions, trying to learn the language of inseminations, donors, pregnancy, and parenting. They were afraid of the pace of the process and worried about a point of "no return." At what point, can you not turn back? At what point are you too far in to call it quits?

Everyone in the group exhaled, breathing into this moment a sigh of recognition and support.

You can press pause whenever you want. You can stop whenever you want to. You can choose how slow you need to go. There is so much that is outside of our control in the process of trying to build our families. It is okay to need to slow down and it is brave to set boundaries.

The group member expressed vulnerable fears about a kind of self-death. What if parenting is the end of who you are, who you were? *It is*, other group members confirmed. You won't be the same and your life will be different. The journey itself is one that requires so much of us — we must learn to communicate our needs in new ways, to understand our relationships in new lights, to plan for future vulnerabilities with children who are their own unique people, outside of our control. "I don't know what it is like for heterosexual people," one group member shared, "but I don't think any of them can understand what *we* go through in this process." Building our family often requires us to learn how to stand up for not only ourselves, our partners, or co-parents, but also for our children or kin. We need to advocate for their needs, their pronouns, their space and autonomy. Our circle grows and our sense of self changes.

And at the end of the day, here is the kicker: You don't need to make a baby to build a family. You don't need to have children in order to call your family complete. Part of building our families is about building relations that don't fall neatly into a cisgender heteronormative vision of futurity, white picket fences, and grandbabies sitting around a dining room table.

Give yourself permission to change course, to press pause, to choose otherwise. Give yourself permission to have even more babies, to keep embryos infinitely on ice, to be a donor, to cherish your kittens and puppies and guinea pigs. Celebrate you and your partners, you and your friendships, you and your kin as more than enough. If this book can teach you your options and help you explore how to communicate your needs, then we have gotten somewhere new together.

Deep breath.

Maybe you got somewhere different than you were expecting, or maybe you are somewhere you always hoped to be. I hope that you can reach your goals and find your people, and if that is not possible, I hope you can feel held and seen in your grief and vulnerability.

It is impossible to imagine how this process will transform you. How loss, sadness, grief, anxiety, and fears can be mixed so closely with elation, excitement, anticipation, and love. We can hold hard and contradictory emotions. We can survive the unexpected celebrations and the challenging surprises. And the truth is that this doesn't always get easier: we feel deep love for the successes and still grieve the losses. We feel unexplainable awe and wonder at what bodies can produce, while still sometimes feeling the weight of what our bodies were unable to do. We feel the happiness and joy of playdates and first words and sadness for the shift in social life.

This isn't easy.

Sometimes it doesn't feel worth it.

These thoughts don't mean your family won't feel complete. These feelings do not mean you will not be a parent. The transformation from who you were into who you are becoming is a product of the hardships of this journey, and that grief and elation can feel complicated and heavy.

The only thing I can promise you is that you are not alone. You are not alone. You are not alone.

Find resources now. Reach out now. Grow community now. We are building a new world together, a new kind of self and new kin and relations, awakening within us the possibilities for new lives, expanding our idea of what family can be.

ACTIVITY

• • •

ULTIMATELY, THE REST OF THE STORY IS YOURS TO TELL

_____

_____

_____

_____

_____

_____

_____

_____

_____

_____

_____

_____

_____

_____

_____

_____

_____

_____

Works Cited

Abdelhakim, A. M., Abd-ElGawad, M., Hussein, R. S., & Abbas, A. M. (2020). Vaginal versus intramuscular progesterone for luteal phase support in assisted reproductive techniques: A systematic review and meta-analysis of randomized controlled trials. *Gynecological Endocrinology, 36*(5), 389–397.

Akuffo-Addo, E., Udounwa, T., Chan, J., & Cauchi, L. (2023). Exploring biologic treatment hesitancy among black and indigenous populations in Canada: A review. *Journal of Racial and Ethnic Health Disparities, 10*(2), 942–951.

Annan, J. J. K., Gudi, A., Bhide, P., Shah, A., & Homburg, R. (2013). Biochemical pregnancy during assisted conception: A little bit pregnant. *Journal of Clinical Medicine Research, 5*(4), 269.

Antonio, M., Lau, F., Davison, K., Devor, A., Queen, R., & Courtney, K. (2022). Toward an inclusive digital health system for sexual and gender minorities in Canada. *Journal of the American Medical Informatics Association, 29*(2), 379–384.

Beshar, I., Deng, J., Alvero, R. J., & Bavan, B. (2021). A decision model predicting the success and cost of IVF using frozen banked versus fresh directed donor oocytes. *Fertility and Sterility, 116*(3), e32.

Bond-Theriault, C. (2024). *Queering reproductive justice: An invitation.* Stanford University Press.

Brushwood Rose, C. T., & Goldberg, S. (2009). *And baby makes more: Known donors, queer parents, and our unexpected families.* Insomniac Press.

Burks, C. A., Purdue-Smithe, A., DeVilbiss, E., Mumford, S., & Weinerman, R. (2024). Frozen autologous and donor oocytes are associated with differences in clinical and neonatal outcomes compared with fresh oocytes: A Society for Assisted Reproductive Technology Clinic Outcome Reporting System Analysis. *F&S Reports, 5*(1), 40–46.

Cattapan, A. (2013). Rhetoric and reality: "Protecting" women in Canadian public policy on assisted human reproduction. *Canadian Journal of Women and the Law, 25*(2), 202–220.

Choudhury, C. A. (2016). New Approaches and Challenges to Reproductive Justice. *FIU Law Review*, 12(1), 1–8.

Cidro, J., Bach, R., & Frohlick, S. (2020). Canada's forced birth travel: Towards feminist indigenous reproductive mobilities. *Mobilities*, 15(2), 173–187.

Comeau, D., Johnson, C., & Bouhamdani, N. (2023). Review of current 2SLGBTQIA+ inequities in the Canadian health care system. *Frontiers in Public Health*, 11, 1183284.

Cranston-Reimer, S. (2019). Reproducing ~~which~~ Nation? White Pro-Natalism and Ontario's Recent Fertility Treatment try Program. *TOPIA: Canadian Journal of Cultural Studies*, 40, 66–87.

Craven, C. (2019). *Reproductive losses: Challenges to LGBTQ family-making.* Routledge.

Craven, C. & Peel, E. (2017). Queering reproductive loss: Exploring grief and memorialization. In E. R. M. Lind & A. Deveau (Eds.), *Interrogating pregnancy loss: Feminist writings on abortion, miscarriage and stillbirth* (pp. 225–245). Demeter Press.

Daniels, C. R., & Golden, J. (2004). Procreative compounds: Popular eugenics, Artificial insemination and the rise of the American sperm banking industry. *Journal of Social History*, 38(1), 5–27.

de Montigny, F., Verdon, C., Meunier, S., Zeghiche, S., Lalande, D. Williams-Plouffe, M. C. (2018). *Supporting families after a perinatal death. Brief presented to the HUMA Committee by the Centre for Studies and Research on Family Intervention and the Canada Research Chair in Family Psychosocial Health.* Gatineau, QC: CERIF/UQO.

de Nie, I., van Mello, N. M., Vlahakis, E., Cooper, C., Peri, A., den Heijer, M., Meibner, A., Huirne, J., & Pang, K. C. (2023). Successful restoration of spermatogenesis following gender-affirming hormone therapy in transgender women. *Cell Reports Medicine*, 4, 100858.

Devine, K., Richter, K. S., Jahandideh, S., Widra, E. A., & McKeeby, J. L. (2021). Intramuscular progesterone optimizes live birth from programmed frozen embryo transfer: A randomized clinical trial. *Fertility and Sterility*, 116(3), 633–643.

Dinshaw, C., et al. (2007). Theorizing queer temporalities: A roundtable discussion. *GLQ: A Journal of Lesbian and Gay Studies*, 13(2), 177–195.

Dorri, A. A., & Russell, S. T. (2022). Future parenting aspirations and minority stress in US sexual minority adults. *Journal of Family Psychology*, 36(7), 1173–1182.

Dwyer, A. (2018). Creating community and creating family: Our QTBIPOC parenting group. In J. Haritaworn, G. Moussa, & S. M. Ware (Eds.), *Marvellous grounds: Queer of colour histories of Toronto*. Between the Lines.

Freeman, E. (2010). *Time binds: Queer temporalities, queer histories*. Duke University Press.

Garbes, A. (2022). *Essential labor: Mothering as social change*. Harper Wave.

Gato, J., Santos, S., & Fontaine, A. M. (2017). To have or not to have children? That is the question. Factors influencing parental decisions among lesbians and gay men. *Sexuality Research and Social Policy, 14*(3), 310–323.

Gill, P., Axelrod, C., Chan, C., & Shapiro, H. (2019). A step towards equitable access: Understanding the use of fertility services by immigrant women in Toronto. *Journal of Obstetrics and Gynecology Canada, 41*(3), 283–291.

Gisondi, M. A., & Bigham, B. (2021). LGBTQ+ health: A failure of medical education. *Canadian Journal of Emergency Medicine, 23*, 577–578.

Goldberg, A. E. (2022). LGBTQ-parent families: Diversity, intersectionality, and social context. *Current Opinion in Psychology*, 101517.

Gregory K. B., Mielke J. G., Neiterman E. (2022). Building families through healthcare: Experiences of lesbians using reproductive services. *Journal of Patient Experience, 9*. doi: 10.1177/23743735221089459.

Gruben, V. (2020). Self-regulation as a means of regulating privately financed medicare: What can we learn from the fertility sector? In C. M. Flood & B. Thomas (Eds.), *Is two-tier health care the future?* (pp. 145–182). University of Ottawa Press.

Halberstam, Jack. (2005). *In a queer time and place: Transgender bodies, subcultural lives*. NYU Press.

Hawthorne, B. (2022). *Raising antiracist children: A practical parenting guide*. Simon & Schuster.

Howat, A., Masterson, C., & Darwin, Z. (2023). Non-birthing mothers' experiences of perinatal anxiety and depression: Understanding the perspectives of the non-birthing mothers in female same-sex parented families. *Midwifery, 120*, 103650.

Ismayilova, M., & Yaya, S. (2023). "I'm usually being my own doctor": Women's experiences of managing polycystic ovary syndrome in Canada. *International Health, 15*(1), 56–66.

Jadva, V. (2021). Sibling relationships across families created through assisted reproduction. In A. Buchanan & A. Rotkirch (Eds.), *Brothers and sisters: Sibling relationships across the life course* (pp. 171–184). Springer.

Jalaliani, S., Davar, R., Akbarzadeh, F., Emami, F., & Eftekhar, M. (2022). Addition of intramuscular to vaginal progesterone for luteal phase support in fresh embryo transfer cycles: A cross-sectional study. *International Journal of Reproductive BioMedicine, 20*(9), 745.

James-Abra, S., Tarasoff, L. A., Green, D., Epstein, R., Anderson, S., Marvel, S., & Ross, L. E. (2015). Trans people's experiences with assisted reproduction services: A qualitative study. *Human Reproduction, 30*(6), 1365–1374.

Kali, L. (2022). *Queer conception: The complete fertility guide for queer and trans parents-to-be.* National Geographic Books.

Karpman, H. E., Ruppel, E. H., & Torres, M. (2018). "It wasn't feasible for us": Queer women of color navigating family formation. *Family Relations, 67*(1), 118–131.

Kennedy, B. (2022). *Good inside: A guide to becoming the parent you want to be.* Harper Wave.

Kennedy, K. B. (2018, March 30). *One hundred (and three) swims.* GUTS, 9. https://gutsmagazine.ca/one-hundred-and-three-swims/.

Kirubarajan, A., Barker, L. C., Leung, S., Ross, L. E., Zaheer, J., Park, B., Abramovich, A., Yudin, M., & Lam, J. S. H. (2022). LGBTQ2S+ childbearing individuals and perinatal mental health: A systematic review. *BJOG: An International Journal of Obstetrics & Gynaecology, 129*(10), 1630–1643.

Kirubarajan, A., Patel, P., Leung, S., Park, B., & Sierra, S. (2021a). Cultural competence in fertility care for lesbian, gay, bisexual, transgender, and queer people: A systematic review of patient and provider perspectives. *Fertility and Sterility, 115*(5), 1294–1301.

Kirubarajan, A., Patel, P., Leung, S., Prethipan, T., & Sierra, S. (2021b). Barriers to fertility care for racial/ethnic minority groups: A qualitative systematic review. *F&S Reviews, 2*(2), 150–159.

Korpaisarn, S., & Safer, J. D. (2018). Gaps in transgender medical education among healthcare providers: A major barrier to care for transgender persons. *Reviews in Endocrine and Metabolic Disorders, 19*(3), 271–275.

Lee, M., Tasa-Vinyals, E., & Gahagan, J. (2021). Improving the LGBTQ2S+ cultural competency of healthcare trainees: Advancing health professional education. *Canadian Medical Education Journal, 12*(1), e7–e20.

Leung, A., Sakkas, D., Pang, S., Thornton, K. & Resetkova, N. (2019). Assisted reproductive technology outcomes in female-to-male transgender patients compared with cisgender patients: A new frontier in reproductive medicine. *Fertility and Sterility, 112*(5), 858–865.

Lien, K., Vujcic, B., & Ng, V. (2021). Attitudes, behaviour, and comfort of Canadian emergency medicine residents and physicians in caring for 2SLGBTQI+ patients. *Canadian Journal of Emergency Medicine*, 23, 617–625.

Mamo, L. (2007). *Queering reproduction: Achieving pregnancy in the age of technoscience.* Duke University Press.

Marshall, K. (2021). *Reproductive rainbow: Exploring fertility intentions and family planning experiences within the 2SLGBTQ community* [Doctoral dissertation, University of Saskatchewan].

Marvel, S. (2016). Laws of conception: A queer genealogy of Canada's Assisted Human Reproduction Act. *FIU Law Review*, 12, 81.

Marvel, S., Tarasoff, L., Epstein, R., Green, D. C., Steele, L., & Ross, L. (2016). Listening to LGBTQ people on assisted human reproduction: Access to reproductive material, services, and facilities. In Trudo Lemmens (Ed.), *Regulating Creation: The Law, Ethics, and Policy of Assisted Human Reproduction* (325–358). University of Toronto Press.

Meyer, I. H. (2015). Resilience in the study of minority stress and health of sexual and gender minorities. *Psychology of sexual orientation and gender diversity*, 2(3), 209.

Minturn, M. S., Martinez, E. I., Le, T., Nokoff, N., Fitch, L., Little, C. E., & Lee, R. S. (2021). Early intervention for LGBTQ health: A 10-hour curriculum for preclinical health professions students. *MedEdPORTAL*, 17, 11072.

Nina, J. L., Zhang, A., Kattari, S., Moravek, M., & Zebrack, B. (2022). "Queer insights": Considerations and challenges for assessing sex, gender identity, and sexual orientation in oncofertility research. *Annals of LGBTQ Public and Population Health.* May. doi:10.1891/LGBTQ-2021-0017.

Ottawa Fertility Centre. (2023, August 3). *Pregnancy loss.* https://conceive.ca/patient-resources/pregnancy-loss/.

Pabuccu, E., Kovanci, E., Israfilova, G., Tulek, F., Demirel, C., & Pabuccu, R. (2022). Oral, vaginal or intramuscular progesterone in programmed frozen embryo transfer cycles: A pilot randomized controlled trial. *Reproductive Biomedicine Online*, 45(6), 1145–1151.

Paynter, M. (2022). *Abortion to abolition: Reproductive health and justice in Canada.* Fernwood Publishing.

Pfeffer, C. A., Hines, S., Pearce, R., Riggs, D. W., Ruspini, E., & White, F. R. (2023). Medical uncertainty and reproduction of the "normal": Decision-making around testosterone therapy in transgender pregnancy. *SSM — Qualitative Research in Health 4*, 100297.

Pirtea, P., De Ziegler, D., Tao, X., Sun, L., Zhan, Y., Ayoubi, J. M., ... & Scott Jr., R. T. (2021). Rate of true recurrent implantation failure is low: Results of three successive frozen euploid single embryo transfers. *Fertility and Sterility, 115*(1), 45–53.

Rachlin, R., and Goodman, M. (2023). *Baby making for everybody: Family building and fertility for LGBTQ+ and solo parents.* Balance.

Romanski, P. A., Aluko, A., Bortoletto, P., Elias, R., & Rosenwaks, Z. (2022). Age-specific blastocyst conversion rates in embryo cryopreservation cycles. *Reproductive BioMedicine Online, 45*(3), 432–439.

Ross, L., & Solinger, R. (2017). *Reproductive justice: An introduction,* Vol. 1. University of California Press.

Ross, L. E., Steele, L. S., & Epstein, R. (2006). Service use and gaps in services for lesbian and bisexual women during donor insemination, pregnancy, and the postpartum period. *Journal of Obstetrics and Gynaecology Canada, 28*(6), 505–511.

Ross, L. J. (2018). Teaching reproductive justice: An activist's approach. In O. N. Perlow, D. I. Wheeler, S. L. Bethea, & B. M. Scott (Eds.), *Black women's liberatory pedagogies: Resistance, transformation, and healing within and beyond the academy* (159–180). Palgrave Macmillan.

Royster, F. T. (2023). *Choosing family: A memoir of queer motherhood and black resistance.* Abrams Press.

Scala, F. (2009). Feminist ideals versus bureaucratic norms: The case of feminist researchers and the Royal Commission on New Reproductive Technologies. In Y. Abu-Laban (Ed.), *Gendering the Nation-State: Canadian and Comparative Perspectives* (97–119). UBC Press.

Scheib, J. E., & Ruby, A. (2008). Contact among families who share the same sperm donor. *Fertility and Sterility, 90*(1), 33–43.

Schreiber, M., Ahmad, T., Scott, M., Imrie, K., & Razack, S. (2021). The case for a Canadian standard for 2SLGBTQIA+ medical education. *CMAJ, 193*(16), E562–E565.

Setti, A. S., Braga, D. P. D. A. F., Iaconelli, A., & Borges, E. (2021). Fresh oocyte cycles yield improved embryo quality compared with frozen oocyte cycles in an egg-sharing donation programme. *Zygote, 29*(3), 234–238.

Sharman, Z. (2021). *The care we dream of: Liberatory and transformative approaches to LGBTQ+ health.* Arsenal Pulp Press.

Shenkman, G., Levy, S., Winkler, Z. B. D., Bass, D., & Geller, S. (2022). Higher levels of postnatal depressive symptomatology, post-traumatic growth, and life satisfaction among gay fathers through surrogacy in comparison to heterosexual fathers: A study in Israel in times of COVID-19. *International Journal of Environmental Research and Public Health*, *19*(13), 7946.

Shufelt, C. L., Torbati, T., & Dutra, E. (2017). Hypothalamic amenorrhea and the long-term health consequences. *Seminars in Reproductive Medicine*, *35*(3), 256–262.

Siegel, D. J. (1999). *The developing mind: Toward a neurobiology of interpersonal experience*. Guilford Press.

Siegel, M., Legler, M., Neziraj, F., Goldberg, A. E., & Zemp, M. (2022). Minority stress and positive identity aspects in members of LGBTQ+ parent families: Literature review and a study protocol for a mixed-methods evidence synthesis. *Children*, *9*(9), 1364.

SisterSong. (2023). "Where did reproductive justice come from?" *Visioning New Futures for Reproductive Justice*. https://docs.google.com/document/d/1ISAq_YXpFW5K7QavUfDQSyxKMuN-JZZ90e9QU1WM4kw/edit.

Smietana, M., Thompson, C., & Twine, F. W. (2018). Making and breaking families — reading queer reproductions, stratified reproduction and reproductive justice together. *Reproductive Biomedicine & Society Online*, *7*, 112.

Standeven, L. R., McEvoy, K. O., & Osborne, L. M. (2020). Progesterone, reproduction, and psychiatric illness. *Best Practice & Research Clinical Obstetrics & Gynaecology*, *69*, 108–126.

Stote, K. (2017). Decolonizing feminism: From reproductive abuse to reproductive justice. *Atlantis: Critical Studies in Gender, Culture & Social Justice/ Études Critiques sur le Genre, la Culture, et la Justice*, *38*(1).

Tam, M. W. (2021). Queering reproductive access: Reproductive justice in assisted reproductive technologies. *Reproductive Health*, *18*, 1–6.

Twine, F. W., & Smietana, M. (2022). The racial contours of queer reproduction. In S. Han & C. Tomori (Eds.), *The Routledge Handbook of Anthropology and Reproduction*. Taylor & Francis.

Weschler, T. (2003). *Taking charge of your fertility: The definitive guide to natural birth control, pregnancy achievement, and reproductive health*. Random House.

World Health Organization. (2023a). *Polycystic ovary syndrome*. World Health Organization. https://www.who.int/news-room/fact-sheets/detail/polycystic-ovary-syndrome#:~:text=Polycystic%20ovary%20syndrome%20(PCOS)%20affects,a%20leading%20cause%20of%20infertility.

World Health Organization. (2023b). *Infertility*. Fact Sheet. https://www.who.int/news-room/fact-sheets/detail/infertility#:~:text=Infertility%20is%20a%20disease%20of,on%20their%20families%20and%20communities.

Xu, H., Zhang, X. Q., Zhu, X. L., Weng, H. N., Xu, L. Q., Huang, L., & Liu, F. H. (2021). Comparison of vaginal progesterone gel combined with oral dydrogesterone versus intramuscular progesterone for luteal support in hormone replacement therapy-frozen embryo transfer cycle. *Journal of Gynecology Obstetrics and Human Reproduction*, 50(7), 102110.

Zafar, A. (2024, April 19). Health Canada lifts policy banning sperm donations from men who have sex with men. C B C *news*. https://cbc.ca/news/health/sperm-donation-health-canada-1.7178631.

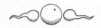

Acknowledgements

Writing this book was a response to both a gap in literature and a personal need to contribute to positive change through knowledge sharing. I have gathered insights from community, from research, from experience, and from conversation. I am grateful to all of those who were part of my learning process and who trusted me to hold their experiences with integrity and care.

To my wife, Joanna, thank you for your patience, your support, your time, and most of all, your unending commitment to communication. It has changed me and shaped so much of how I approach fertility, care, and relationships in this book and in my daily life. You continue to teach me how to share, be vulnerable, express needs, and be honest with myself and others. Your transparency and openness is brave and contagious. I am so privileged to build a family with you.

To Tanya and Jazz, thank you. Thank you. Thank you. Your notes, your questions, your guidance and insights have been critical in creating the most inclusive, comprehensive, and clear guide for our diverse 2SLGBTQ+ communities. With each suggestion and comment you pushed me to surprise myself, to consider equity and social justice, and to ensure that the book answered the questions so many community members are asking. Jenn, thank you for your meticulous copyedits. Lauren, thank you for your patience and incredible care in bringing the illustrations and the text together. From the marketing team to layout and communications, everyone on the Fernwood team truly shared with me the urgent desire to bring this book to 2SLGBTQ+ communities.

To Kelsy Vivash, you bring this book to life with elegance, creativity, humour, and love. It is such a privilege to work with you and have you illustrate and draw this journey. I am so appreciative not only for your beautiful artistic creations, but also for our friendship. I can't wait to see what the future holds for our collaborations!

To the contributors of this book, I am so honoured to be in conversation with you. From our first meetings on Zoom, to discuss the need to bring this book into the world, to the beautiful text and interviews you contributed to the book, I am grateful for the opportunity to share, learn, and transform together.

To Birth Mark and Seed and Sprout, thank you for supporting so many queer and transgender parents and families. Thank you for ensuring equitable fertility, pregnancy, and postpartum care, for improving access, valuing lives, and listening to needs. Your work and presence have provided me with a foundation for what reproductive care can and should be. And to Planting the Seed families, thank you for sharing your stories, being drivers of change, showing up and supporting 2SLGBTQ+ family building in new and exciting ways, and cultivating the communities we dream of and so deeply deserve.

To my postdoctoral supervisor, Nathan Lachowsky at the University of Victoria, thank you for your support over the last two years. I am grateful for the incredible opportunities to contribute to research projects at the university and the Community-Based Research Centre that will improve 2SLGBTQ+ reproductive and sexual care and access.

To Alex Wells, thanks for the title, the friendship, and constant support and kindness. I am lucky to have you as a friend, collaborator, and creative inspiration.

Mom, this book has come from the belief you instilled in me (and that your father instilled in you): we can indeed make the world a more just and beautiful place. I am so grateful to learn from your activism, fierce feminism, and love. David, thank you for being the most attentive stepdad and zayde, and for showing such a sincere interest in this work. Bailey, you have forever been my role model, my teacher, and my best friend. I watch you parent and learn the important balance of love, boundaries, poetry, and play. Thank you for helping me navigate hard journeys and always always being my person. Rhonda, having an honorary mother taught me that all families look different and that they don't depend on blood relations. Thank you for inspiring me to be critical and to question, and of course, for showing me how to watch scary movies.

Writing this book has given me the opportunity to read other books, websites, community resources, and social media posts from 2SLGBTQ+ community members, families, and intended parents. Thank you to all of those who continue to share their knowledge and experiences and for allowing me to join the chorus of strong queer voices making a difference.

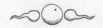

Contributor Bios

LAINE HALPERN ZISMAN is a fertility support practitioner, lecturer, and adjunct assistant professor at the School of Public Health and Social Policy at the University of Victoria, where she completed a post-doctoral fellowship in 2024. She is founder and project lead on a new 2SLGBTQ+ family-building online platform, Family Building Canada (familybuildingcanada.com). Her research traverses the intersections of 2SLGBTQ+ equity, culture, and reproductive care. She has published two collected volumes, *Women and Popular Culture in Canada* (2020) and the second edition of *Queerly Canadian*, co-edited with professor Scott Rayter (2023). Laine received a SSHRC Partner Engage Grant (2023) and SSHRC Connection Grant (2022) to support activities related to HIV *In My Day* at the University of Victoria; she is also the recipient of a CIHR Health Hub fellowship (2022); the CATR O'Neill Book Prize (2022); a Graduate Mellon Fellowship (2017); and the Course Instructor Teaching Excellence Award (2018).

KELSY VIVASH is a queer artist, designer, and writer currently living in Toronto with her spouse and their beloved pets. Her work is inspired by nature and nostalgia, and her artistic training comes almost entirely from fidgeting with Microsoft Paint.

ANNA BALAGTAS (SHE/THEY) is a Filipina queer, non-binary femme radical birthworker, reproductive justice advocate, educator, and community organizer. Their practice is rooted in queer decolonial carework and the prioritization of QTBIPGM wellness, equity, and abundance. They are the founder of Pocket Doula, co-founder of the National Collaboration for Doula Access, and director of Cornerstone Birthwork Canada.

REESE CARR is a queer and trans PhD candidate in women and gender studies at the University of Toronto. Their work focuses on kinship, reproductive politics, care economies, and queer and trans identity formation through state documentation. In 2022, they were awarded a doctoral Canada Graduate Scholarship for their proposed work on the desired and imagined kinship structures of young queer adults in Ontario, as shaped by social movements and policy. Reese also currently works as a researcher and co-producer on the Gender Playground podcast from Witch, Please! Productions. When they aren't surrounded by piles of books, Reese can be found tending their vegetable garden, and throwing clay at their local pottery studio.

SARA COHEN, LLB, is a fertility law lawyer based in Toronto, Ontario. She regularly acts for intended parents, surrogates, donors, cryobanks, hospitals, distributors, and fertility clinics on a wide range of fertility law issues. Sara was named by *Canadian Lawyer* magazine as one of the top 25 most influential lawyers in Canada, by Lexpert as a leading lawyer to watch and won the Precedent Setter Award given by *Precedent Magazine*. She sits on the ethics committee of one of Canada's pre-eminent clinics and is a director of the Canadian Fertility and Andrology Society. She is the past president of Fertility Matters Canada, a former adjunct professor of reproductive law at Osgoode Hall Law School, and a fellow of the Academy of Adoption and

Assisted Reproduction Attorneys. Sara has given expert testimony on third-party reproduction and legal parentage issues and has been invited by the Ontario, Canadian, and Irish governments to provide expert opinions on various fertility and parentage-related legislation. Sara loves what she does and cares deeply about her clients and about mentoring the next generation of Canadian fertility lawyers.

RACHEL EPSTEIN (PHD ED) is a longtime 2SLGBTQ+ parenting activist, educator, and researcher and was the founding coordinator of the LGBTQ Parenting Network in Toronto. She is the editor of the 2009 anthology *Who's Your Daddy? And Other Writings on Queer Parenting* and in 2014 completed a doctoral dissertation on 2SLGBTQ+ people's experiences in fertility clinics. From 2015 to 2017 Rachel was a Banting postdoctoral fellow at Brock University, conducting research on 2SLGBTQ+ family conflict and reconfiguration. She grew up in a secular Jewish household filled with politics, social justice, and music. Her work and activist life have also included ten years working with migrant domestic workers and five years as executive director of a community-based secular Jewish organization. Rachel has facilitated hundreds of workshops for community organizations as well as health, education, and legal professionals and currently works as a facilitator, mediator, fertility counsellor and coach, and wedding officiant. She also recently make a film called *The Anarchist Lunch*.

GABRIELLE GRIFFITH is a gender-nonconforming birth parent, community researcher, educator, and organizer. They serve as a full-spectrum doula, advocating for community care in perinatal mental health. Embracing their identities as Black, queer, and disabled, Gabrielle aims to drive change through a queer reproductive justice lens, prioritizing support for QTBIPOC perinatal communities.

BRITT KERNEN graduated with a nursing degree in 2012 and has always had a passion for helping others. Despite starting their career in cardiology, they eventually found their way into fertility nursing, which aligned with Britt's goal to provide client-centred care while making a difference in people's lives. After working at various clinics and growing professionally, they eventually co-founded Fertility for You. They currently work as a nurse team lead at Twig Fertility in Toronto. Ultimately, they strive to provide care that improves patient experiences and ensure that every patient feels supported through their journey.

A.J. LOWIK is an assistant professor at the University of Lethbridge, Department of Sociology. Their research and activism focuses on trans people's reproductive lives and health, and they work to ensure that everyone has access to gender-affirming reproductive healthcare. They are the president of the Abortion Rights Coalition of Canada. A.J. loves knitting, board games, cats, and gardening. They are an unapologetic feminist and queer liberationist.

Index